KV-013-695

DOCTOR, DOCTOR

DR. PETER ROWAN

KINGSTON COLLEGE OF FURTHER EDUCATION
LIBRARY

London: HMSO

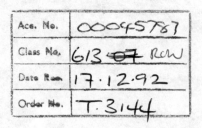

Acc. No.	00045787
Class No.	613 07 Rew
Date Rec.	17.12.92
Order No.	T.3144

Devised and produced by Complete Editions

Illustrations by Susannah English and Harry Venning
Cover Illustration by Susannah English

© Dr Peter Rowan 1992
Applications for reproduction should be made to HMSO
First published 1992

ISBN 0 11 701695 0

HMSO gratefully acknowledges the assistance given by the
Children's Hospital, Birmingham in the preparation of this book.

British Library Cataloguing in Publication Data

A CIP Catalogue record for this book is
available from the British Library

Contents

To Wills and Andrée Gardner

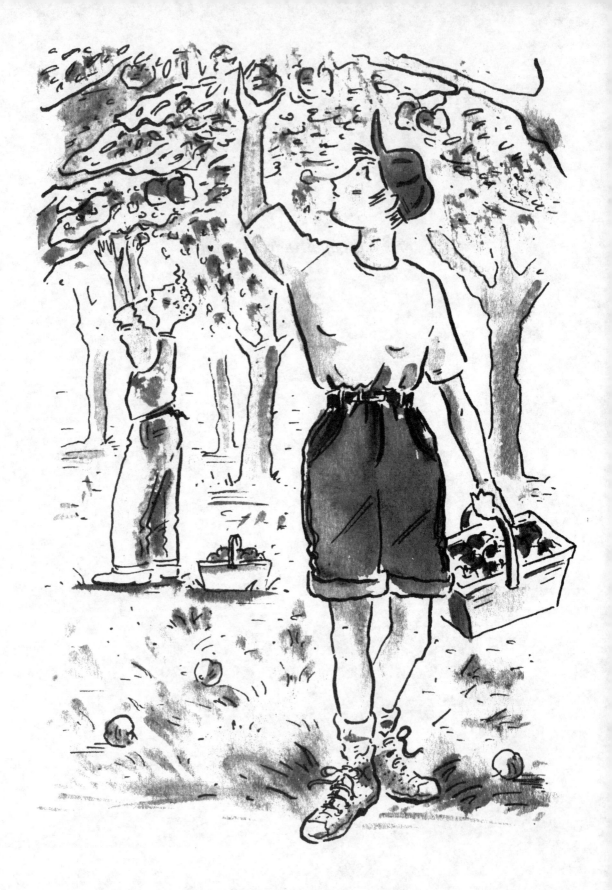

Introduction

All living creatures have eight things in common. Your body is no exception. It's made of cells, it moves, it feeds, it grows, it breathes, it excretes, it's sensitive to the world around it, and it reproduces. That's what this book is all about.

Chapter 1 looks at the human body and these eight characteristics.

Chapter 2 then focuses on reproduction. This perfectly normal part of life is often somehow considered different to these other seven distinctive features of living organisms.

There is so much ignorance and so many fears about 'reproduction', or sex, or intercourse, or whatever you like to call the business of ensuring that the human race continues. The only difference is that sex can be so much more pleasurable than some of the other actions of living organisms.

Chapter 3 is about a ninth thing the body can do – that is to go wrong. This chapter deals with the problems that concern teenagers. Most medical things that might worry you are here.

Chapter 4 is also about things that can affect the health of young people. 'All in the mind' is a neat phrase, but like many neat phrases it doesn't accurately sum up illness, since it's well recognized that the functions of the body and mind are inextricably linked. Mental illnesses such as depression are being recognized more and more in young people.

School days may not, after all, be the happiest days of your life.

So chapter 5 is about people like me who try to help other people who are sick. At one time doctors were not only revered in an almost mystical way, but what they said and did was accepted without question. Nowadays there is an increasing wish to know why and how doctors are treating us. This chapter aims to explain what is happening when you visit your doctor.

Chapter 6 is about the workings of hospitals. Most of us will need the attentions of someone or something within a hospital at some stage of our lives.

Chapter 7 is about First Aid. There

may well be times when you can help someone in trouble before expert help arrives.

Although there is certainly not 'a pill for every ill' there are a lot of different treatments to get different people with different illnesses better – you'll find out about them in Chapter 8.

Chapter 9 is about aspects of world health. While you are reading this thousands of people will have been born and will die before their time. As we approach the year 2000 everyone who can should work towards good health for the whole world.

Now you've got an idea of what's to follow read on and put some flesh on these bones!

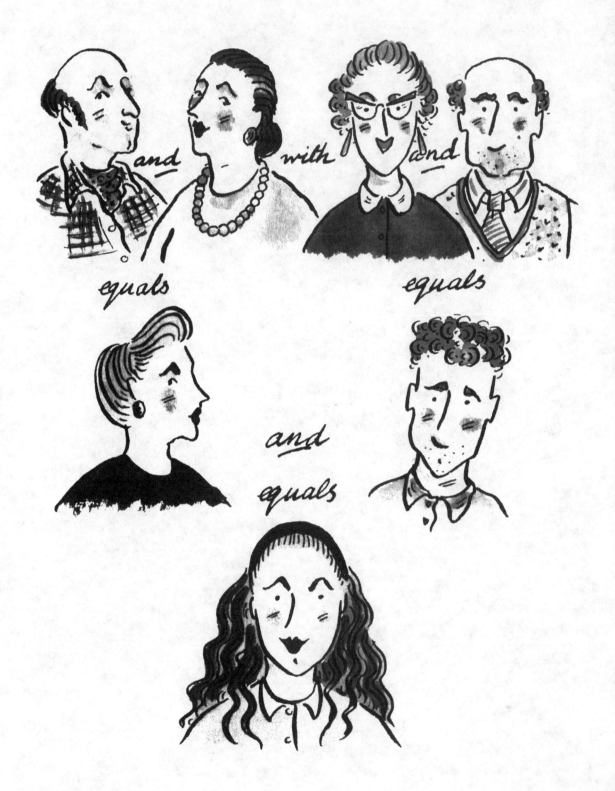

CHAPTER 1

Bodyworks

The human body is an amazing collection of different tissues and organs. The basic building block of these is the cell. Cells come in all sorts of shapes and sizes, and when put together make up the different parts of the body. Thus there are brain cells, bone cells, muscle cells, and blood cells. Each of the systems below is made up of them.

A typical cell is mostly water and is surrounded by a thin cell wall. In the centre is the cell nucleus. If each cell is like a small city, then the nucleus is the city hall. It contains the genetic code in forty-six chromosomes. They are the blueprint for how the body is to be.

The chromosomes are made of millions of genes which are strung together like a strand of beads. The only cells in the body which do not have forty-six chromosomes are the mother's egg (ovum) and the father's sperm. They each have twenty-three, but when combined to produce a living cell, will give the final forty-six.

This means that we all have characteristics from both our mother and father. And, of course, we also have links through our parents to our grandparents. These include obvious features such as hair and eye colour, through to less obvious ones such as tendency to some diseases. These are all inherited from our parents' genes.

In addition to these genes, the food we eat and how we take care of our bodies through such things as exercise, will determine how we look and behave when fully grown.

Brain and Nerves

The nervous system is made up of the brain, nerves and the spinal cord. The brain is like a powerful computer. It is the control tower of the body. The spinal cord is a continuation of this nervous tissue, and runs out of the skull within the protective bones of the spine.

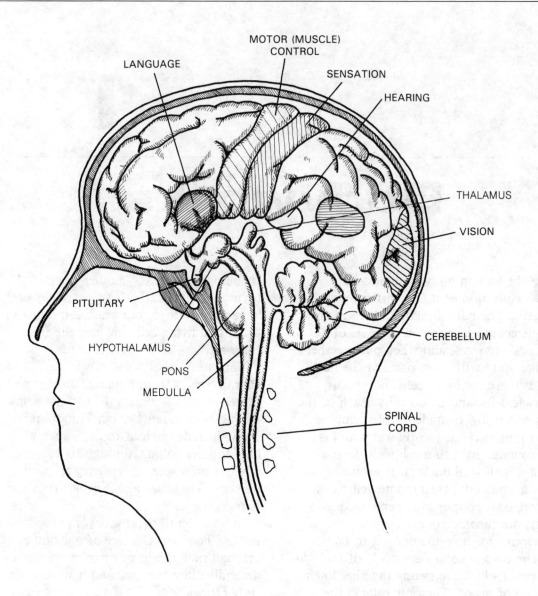

LANGUAGE

MOTOR (MUSCLE) CONTROL

SENSATION

HEARING

THALAMUS

VISION

CEREBELLUM

SPINAL CORD

MEDULLA

PONS

HYPOTHALAMUS

PITUITARY

Cerebrum

This is the most highly evolved and important part of the brain. It is large compared with the size of the rest of the body, and is housed in two halves, or hemispheres, under the top and front of the skull. The left hemisphere tends to

control the right side of the body and the right hemisphere tends to control the left side of the body.

The cerebrum controls conscious thought. Suppose you see someone at a dance that you rather like the look of. Your eyes tell the cerebrum what he or she looks like. The nose may register a pleasant smell if you are close enough.

Brain cells within the cerebrum decide on a positive reaction to all this information. They consciously command the leg muscles to walk over; and having done that they order the muscles involved in speech to ask that person for a dance. The cerebrum, with the aid of the ears, listens to their voice to get more information! It may even order the hands to touch and gather more information through the touch, heat, and vibration receptors in the skin of the finger tips.

If you later fell in love with that person, that too would be cerebrum controlled. This part of the brain houses your ideas, your loves and hates and in fact all your feelings. Memory and language are also stored within its billions of cells.

Cerebellum

The cerebellum of the brain keeps the balance and co-ordination of the body running smoothly. Unlike many of the actions controlled by the cerebrum, the cerebellum acts without you having to think about such functions. Information on the position of the body is continually coming into the cerebellum from the eyes, ears and muscles and is used to keep the body on course like an ocean-going yacht. Next time you run down stairs just note how much conscious thought goes into the movement and control of your legs. Very little. In fact if you start to think about all the actions and influence them at a conscious level you may fall over! The cerebellum is very good at control of these sorts of actions, and does not need

interference from higher centres like the cerebrum.

Thalamus

This relay station in the brain receives the feeling of pain, (as well as some other sensations). It can pass these onto the cerebrum, but may deal with them itself. Thus the pain may not get any further into the brain, and is never 'appreciated' higher up in the cerebrum.

Hypothalamus and pituitary gland

The hypothalamus controls the release of many chemical messengers (hormones) from the pituitary gland. It's involved in essential day to day running of the body through such feelings as thirst and hunger. It also helps regulate the body's temperature.

Mid-brain, pons and medulla

Lower areas of the brain such as the mid-brain, pons, and medulla are a relay station for messages travelling up the spinal cord. Actions such as breathing and the heart beat are controlled here. So when asking that person for a dance, if you felt slightly nervous it would be the medulla which gave you a dry mouth and made the heart beat faster.

Spinal cord

This white rope-like cable runs through holes in the bones of the spine. Sensory nerves run to it bringing information from the body, and motor nerves run out from it carrying messages from the brain.

Some actions are controlled at spinal cord level. The higher parts of the brain don't need to be involved. This is quite handy as these sorts of reflex actions are very fast. If you stand on a nail your foot is moved swiftly off without the need to ask the brain's permission.

Heart and Blood

The heart is a living double-barrelled pump. One side pumps blood rich in oxygen around the body. The other side receives the blood as it returns from the journey, and pumps it to the lungs to be re-oxygenated. This re-oxygenated blood

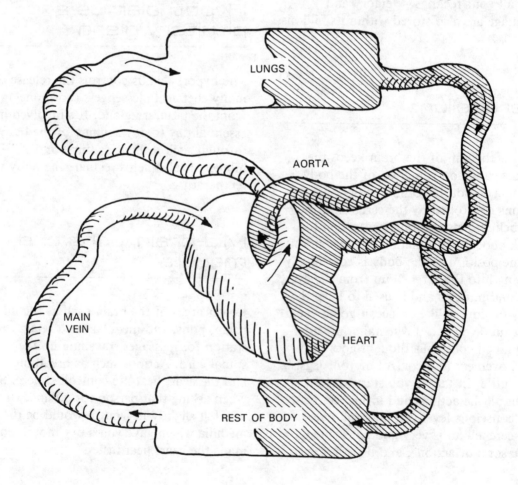

LUNGS

AORTA

MAIN VEIN

HEART

REST OF BODY

then returns to the heart to be pumped around the body again.

Arteries carry oxygenated blood away from the heart. Veins carry it back. Capillaries are fine hair-like blood vessels which are too small to be seen without a microscope. They are the link between the larger arteries and veins. One red blood cell can just squeeze through a capillary. It is at this stage that oxygen leaves the blood to be taken up by the various tissues of the body. It is also the stage where waste products like carbon dioxide are picked up by the circulating blood, and are taken back to the lungs to be released as air is breathed out.

There are about five litres of blood in a fully grown human body. The heart pumps about seventy times per minute at rest, and each day the blood will circulate around the body many hundreds of times.

Blood consists of a straw-coloured fluid (plasma) with cells floating in this soup-like mixture. Most of these are red cells − hence the colour of blood. There are white cells as well to fight infection, and small platelets which help blood clot if you cut yourself. If you're into trivia your circulation has some memorable facts and figures. If all the blood vessels in the body were laid end to end they would reach more than twice around the world − 96,000 km. Capillaries are so small that if one could be made to leak blood into a cup, it would take a hundred years to fill that cup. Each blood cell lives about 120 days before it is replaced. There are 5,000,000 red blood cells in a pin-prick of blood. When it dies a red cell will have made about 172,000 voyages around the body. A typical journey around the body takes a red cell less than one minute.

Lungs and Breathing

The lungs are like two pink rugby balls, and they are set in the chest either side of the heart. They fill with air about twelve times every minute when the body is at rest. The rib cage and the flat muscle called the diaphragm under it act like a large bellows.

The reason that the body needs air from breathing is to bring oxygen into it. All animals need oxygen to live. Blood takes oxygen away from the lungs and the heart pumps it to the tissues. What happens next is very simple. The oxygen burns, or oxidizes, food stuffs that have been brought into the body by the process of digestion. This 'fire' gives off energy and provides the energy to keep body cells working. Using words like 'fire' and 'burn' could mislead anyone who expected to see a rush of energy. This body process of oxidation, or combustion, or burning − call it what you like − is a slow one. So it doesn't appear as suddenly or fiercely as the smoke and flames in a grate. It is just as well that this energy is released at a slow and controlled rate in the body. There is enough energy in a big meal such as steak and chips to cause a fatal rise in body temperature if all the calories were released at once!

Just as the lungs bring oxygen into the

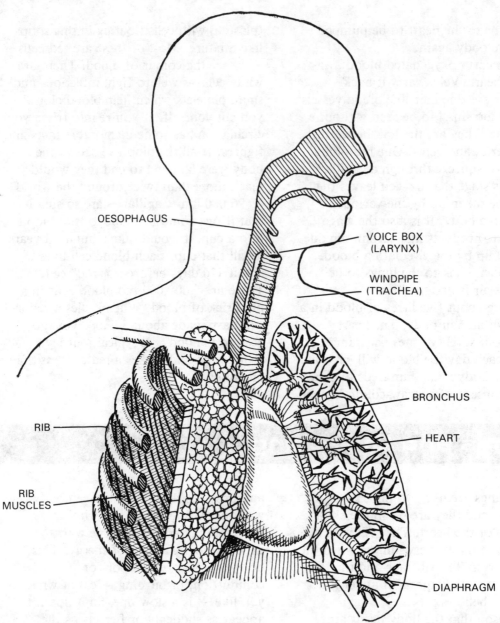

OESOPHAGUS

VOICE BOX
(LARYNX)

WINDPIPE
(TRACHEA)

BRONCHUS

RIB

HEART

RIB
MUSCLES

DIAPHRAGM

body so they take carbon dioxide out. This is the waste product of the combustion. Carbon dioxide and oxygen pass each other in the lungs like passengers getting on and off a train.

Air coming in and out of the lungs is involved in a variety of familiar processes. As air passes between the vocal cords

sounds are produced. We learn to turn these into speech. A cough is an explosion of air out of the lungs which can clear any blockage. A sneeze is a similar act through the nose. A yawn is a slow deep breath. Here's another nugget of trivia. When you sneeze the air leaves the lungs at the speed of a hurricane!

Intestines and Digestive System

Digestion of food begins in the mouth. Teeth cut, chop and grind food into small pieces, as saliva from three pairs of glands pours in to make the food easier to swallow. Saliva also begins the process of food breakdown. When the

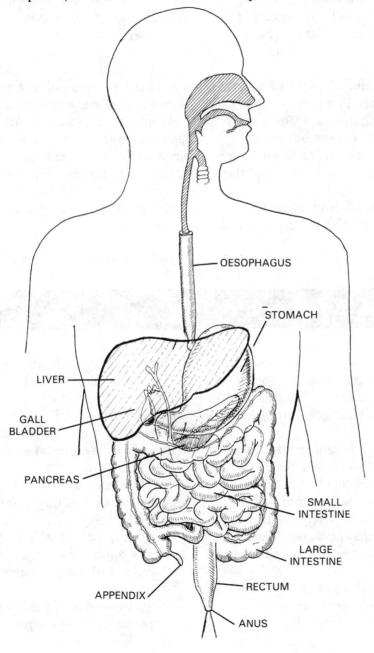

OESOPHAGUS

STOMACH

LIVER

GALL BLADDER

PANCREAS

SMALL INTESTINE

LARGE INTESTINE

RECTUM

APPENDIX

ANUS

food has been chewed, muscles of the mouth and tongue position it correctly, and then throw it backwards into the pharynx from where it travels down the *gullet* (oesophagus) to the stomach.

Once in the *stomach* the food is churned and mixed with more digestive juices and strong hydrochloric acid. The stomach is a widest part of the digestive tube which stretches from the mouth to the anus.

The long coiled tube after the stomach is the small intestine. This area is about six metres long. The walls are 'fluffy' with millions of tiny projections called villi. These enable most of the absorption of food to take place in this section of the bowel.

Into the first part of this tubing (the *duodenum*) more digestive juices pour in from the liver, gall bladder and pancreas gland.

The journey that the food is making is powered by muscular contractions in the walls of the bowel. These squeeze the mushy mashed up food along in a way not unlike the action of toothpaste being squeezed out of a toothpaste tube.

The *large intestine* receives what's left of the food, and a slower journey begins along this wider tube. By now the 'food' is a watery mixture and as it passes along much of the water is absorbed out.

About one to two days after the meal has been eaten the unwanted, nearly solid, waste arrives at the end of the bowel. At a convenient moment, and hopefully in a convenient place, the muscles of the *rectum* push the waste matter (faeces) out of the *anus*.

Immune System

The body has a self-defence system. Without it the human body would soon fall victim to serious ill health and even death. (This is what goes wrong in AIDS.)

Blood contains white cells, made in the bone marrow and also in the lymph glands, and these can engulf, for example, unwanted bacteria. You have probably already felt these glands after a bad sore throat. They swell up like castles bulging with an increased garrison of troops ready for a good fight.

Some white cells also produce proteins called antibodies. The immune system is capable of producing thousands of different types of antibodies, and these may be tailor-made to combat the known threat of a particular virus.

This system is well illustrated by what happens when a vaccination against German measles (rubella) is given.

1. To vaccinate against German measles a live version of the virus is injected into the body.
2. The immune system is stimulated and forms antibodies against German measles without producing the actual illness.
3. Sometime later, if the body is exposed to the real virus, these

antibodies are released like a pack of fierce dogs into the blood stream and they will kill the German measles virus. The body itself comes to no harm, and its owner will probably not notice that anything has happened.

Skin

The body is clothed by the largest human organ, the skin, which has a number of functions.

1. About sixty per cent of the human body is water, yet it has to survive on dry land. The skin has a large part to

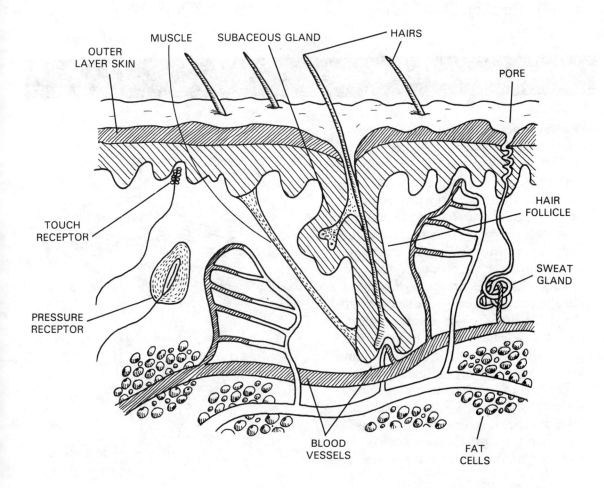

OUTER
LAYER SKIN

MUSCLE

SUBACEOUS GLAND

HAIRS

PORE

TOUCH
RECEPTOR

HAIR
FOLLICLE

PRESSURE
RECEPTOR

SWEAT
GLAND

BLOOD
VESSELS

FAT
CELLS

play in this, keeping a precise water balance between the body and the environment. The skin keeps body water in, and also keeps excess water out when the body gets wet.

2. It holds nerve endings that register sensations like touch, heat, cold and pain.

3. It controls body temperature. If the environment gets hot, glands in the skin release sweat. This evaporates into the air, and takes excess body heat with it. In a cooler environment blood may be withdrawn from the skin into the deeper tissues of the body, and heat can be conserved.

4. Skin protects the body from such things as germs, dirt and the sun's rays.

5. Skin plays a part in nutrition. Some vitamin D is made in the skin when sunlight falls on it.

Toe nails and finger nails are special parts of skin. They grow out from a root. As with hair, they have no nerves so it doesn't hurt to cut them. Hair grows out of skin in a similar way to nails. The hair follicle is the pit from which the hair grows. The follicle shape determines if the hair is naturally straight, curly or wavy. Hair colour depends on what pigment melanin is in the hair. This pigment also determines the skin colour.

Kidneys and Water

The exact amount of water in the human body has to be kept within strict limits. Water comes in with food and drink, and is also made by the body's cells as part of the energy producing process. It also goes out of the body. The most obvious route is via the two kidneys, which are constantly filtering the blood and removing waste products. The separated waste – products of body metabolism like urea – are sent out in the yellow liquid which amongst other names is called urine. The urine is stored in a muscular bag – the bladder – until with luck you are near a toilet.

The kidneys are able to control body water. If you drink a lot, more diluted urine is made to get rid of this excess fluid. On a hot dry day when the body is sweating a minimum of urine is produced

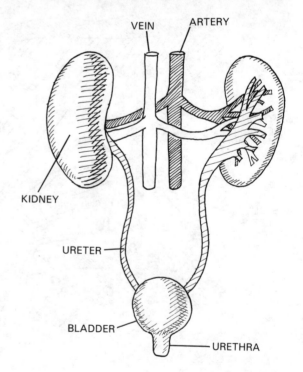

to save water. Some is lost from the body in sweat, and in air breathed out of the lungs. A little is lost down the toilet when you have your bowels open, and a very small amount is lost in tears from the eyes.

Bones, muscles, ligaments, and joints

The framework of the body are the 206 or so bones. These are the scaffolding on which everything else hangs. Many of the joints between bones are linked by ligaments, and many have muscles attached to them by tendons. Contraction of a muscle will move a joint.

So the biceps flexes the elbow and the triceps extends it. These are muscles under voluntary control. Other muscles – for example the heart – work automatically.

Bones are also hard and protective. The brain is protected inside the skull.

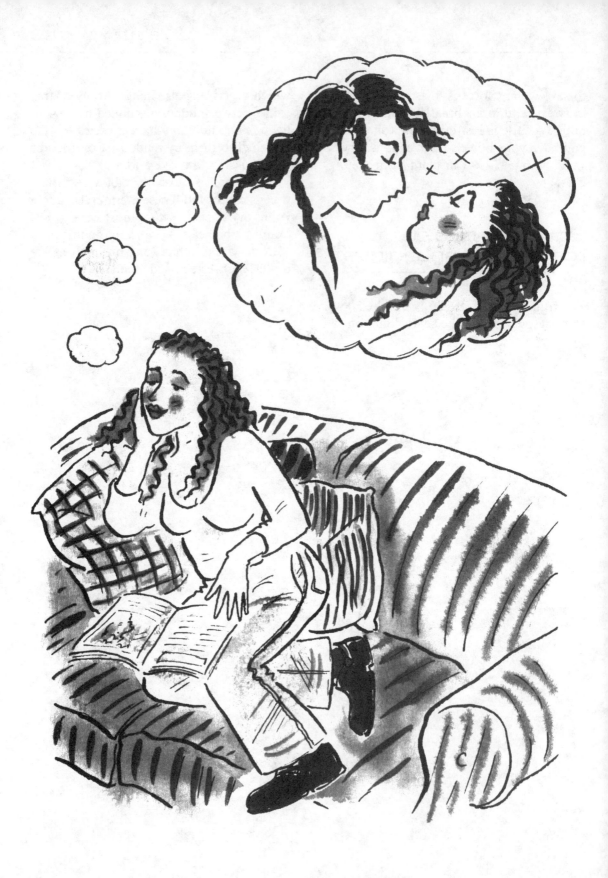

2

The Beginners Guide to Sex

Puberty, or adolescence as it's also called, is a time when your body changes from that of a child into that of an adult. It starts as chemical messengers are released from the brain. They trigger other chemicals called hormones from the ovaries and testicles, and these produce changes in the growing body.

This can be a strain emotionally for all concerned. The young person has to cope with powerful and sometimes confusing physical and mental changes, which parents have to adjust to as well. Common sense on both sides can smooth over a difficult time.

There is no set pattern for all the changes that take place. Each individual person 'grows up' at a different speed, and in their own way . The end result is the same though − a healthy fully developed adult by the age of eighteen.

At the age of ten boys and girls are of a very similar general build. By fifteen many physical changes will have taken place.

Boys are taller and more muscular than girls, who have developed breasts and become more 'curvy' as body fat develops around hips and thighs. Boys' shoulders are more muscular.

As you have probably noticed boys and girls are constructed slightly differently! Most of the male organs are visible − with clothes off − whilst most of the female ones are hidden within the lower part of the abdomen.

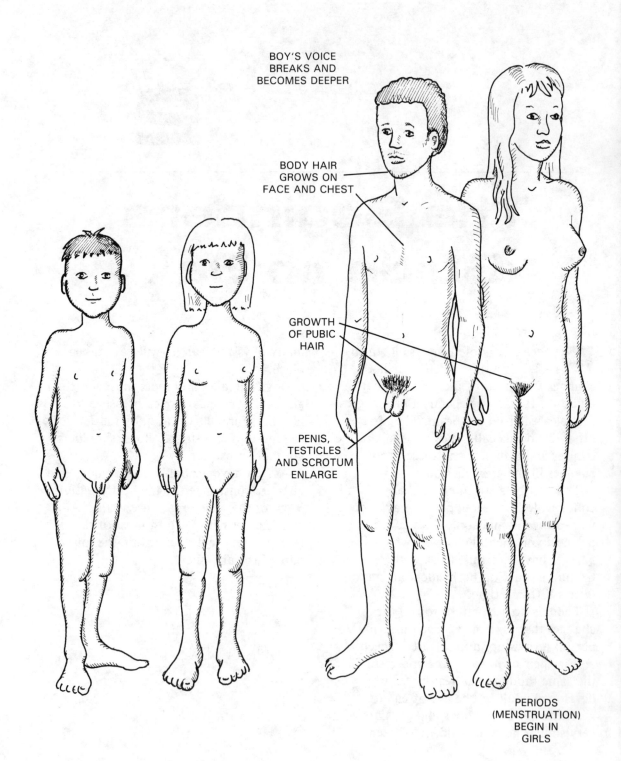

BOY'S VOICE
BREAKS AND
BECOMES DEEPER

BODY HAIR
GROWS ON
FACE AND CHEST

GROWTH
OF PUBIC
HAIR

PENIS,
TESTICLES
AND SCROTUM
ENLARGE

PERIODS
(MENSTRUATION)
BEGIN IN
GIRLS

Male sex organs

Penis

The penis, cock, willy, 'one eyed trouser snake', percy, or whichever of its many other nicknames you use, is formed from three columns of erectile tissue. Its tip is enlarged to form the glans of the penis. The foreskin (prepuce) covers the end of the glans. This is sometimes surgically removed (circumcision) for religious or health reasons. Boys who have not been circumcised should be able to roll the foreskin back to wash underneath it.

A tube (urethra) passes through the penis down which urine can run out of the bladder. Semen also shoots out of here during ejaculation.

Erections occur as the three columns within the penis fill up with blood. Arteries pump them up, while veins are compressed by muscles, so the blood can't flow out of the penis.

Although the penis grows in size during puberty, it almost never ends up big enough to satisfy its owner. A lot of men get very worried that they have a smaller penis than others. There are two things to say about this:

1. There's nothing you can do to get a bigger one.
2. Once erect, penises are more or less the same size, whatever they looked like before.

Testicle

Like its counterpart the ovary, the testicle or testis, or ball, or bollock (among its commonest names) has two basic

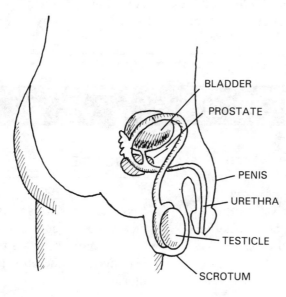

BLADDER

PROSTATE

PENIS

URETHRA

TESTICLE

SCROTUM

functions. It produces sperm and it produces the hormones which bring about the body changes that turn a boy into a man and keeps him that way.

Sperm

Sperm is made within each of the two testicles as they lie within a bag of skin called the scrotum. Testicles hang outside the body because a temperature lower than that of the body's is necessary for sperm development. A system of connecting tubes delivers the sperm to the outside world via the penis.

There are millions of sperm in each ejaculate. They are supported by a milky white liquid which is secreted by a gland at the base of the bladder. Sperm and this fluid are called semen. The sperm 'swim' a distance of about ten centimetres to meet the female's ovum. They do this at a speed of eighteen centimetres per hour. If looked at under a miscroscope they can be seen wriggling like tadpoles. A sperm is much smaller than an ovum. Forty sperm could lie end-to-end across the head of a pin, but an ovum is just visible to the naked eye, measuring about an eighth of a millimetre in diameter.

Boys may have what are called 'wet dreams'. They ejaculate or 'come' during the night and find their pyjamas wet in the morning. Again there is nothing wrong if this happens.

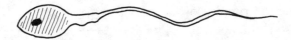

Many boys and girls relieve sexual tension by masturbating. This is defined as stimulating the genitals without intercourse to produce an orgasm — the intense and pleasurable sensation at the climax of sexual excitement. There are a lot of myths about this harmless practice. It will not cause blindness, or any other form of ill health.

Female Sex Organs

The vulvae are the visible parts of the female sex organs. They comprise two lips, or labia. These lips cover the opening of the vagina, as well as the outlet from the bladder, and a sensitive area of tissue called the clitoris.

Vagina

Like the penis, this is known by plenty of nicknames — cunt and fanny are two of the commonest. It's a muscular tube leading from the outside world to the uterus.

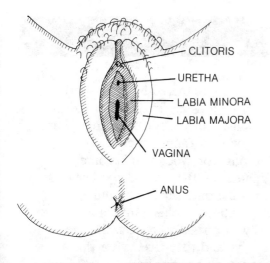

Ovary

There is an ovary on each side of the body and each is about the same size as a testicle. At birth each ovary contains about 3,000,000 ova. Less than one in 15,000 of these will be shed each month during life.

Uterus

Also called the womb, the uterus is a pear shaped muscular cavity, whose neck is called the cervix, and is connected to the vagina.

Fallopian tubes

One on each side, they run from the womb to the ovaries.

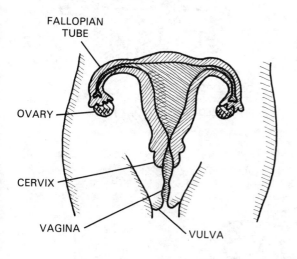

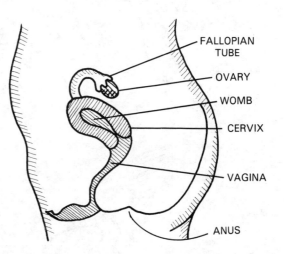

A virgin is someone who has not had sexual intercourse. In *some* girls who are virgins there is a thin membrane across part of the vagina. This is called the hymen.

Periods

Girls usually have their first period sometime between the ages of nine and sixteen. It varies so do not worry if your friend 'starts' before you. If you haven't had one by the age of sixteen get some advice from your doctor.

There is usually a small amount of bleeding at first. You'll notice this on your pants.

After a year or so the periods will settle down to a monthly (twenty-eight day) cycle – that's why, along with the curse, being on the blob and other names, it's also called the monthly.

If you are bothered by heavy periods, or your periods are irregular or painful, then you could ask for help from your Mum, or your family doctor.

Periods stop when you become pregnant. But there are also other reasons for missing one, such as an illness, moving house or changing school. Periods usually stop finally between the ages of forty-five and fifty-five. After this a woman can't become pregnant.

Some girls have painful periods. There are effective treatments for this, so ask for advice from your mother or your

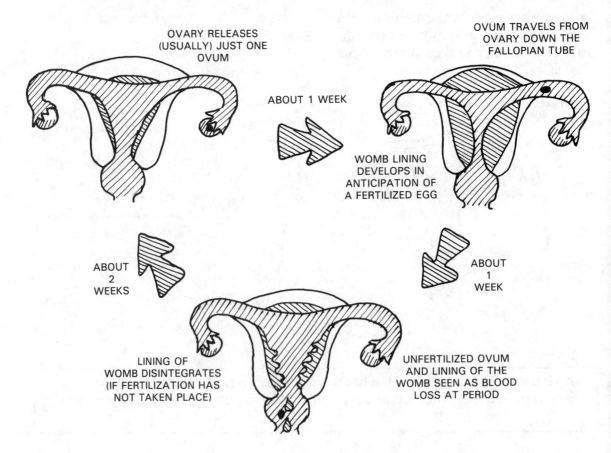

OVARY RELEASES (USUALLY) JUST ONE OVUM

ABOUT 1 WEEK

OVUM TRAVELS FROM OVARY DOWN THE FALLOPIAN TUBE

WOMB LINING DEVELOPS IN ANTICIPATION OF A FERTILIZED EGG

ABOUT 2 WEEKS

ABOUT 1 WEEK

LINING OF WOMB DISINTEGRATES (IF FERTILIZATION HAS NOT TAKEN PLACE)

UNFERTILIZED OVUM AND LINING OF THE WOMB SEEN AS BLOOD LOSS AT PERIOD

doctor. Some girls feel a bit down, moody or irritable before a period. This goes when the period starts.

During the period a girl may choose to wear a sanitary towel on the outside of the body, or an internal tampon. These are all disposable, and as you will change them frequently and wash, there will be no smell. In fact, as you cannot see them, no one will know you have a period unless you tell them.

Having a period is *not* an illness. It is a normal part of a woman's life. You can wash your hair and have a bath during a period. It is important to stay fresh and clean. Exercise is fine too. If you want to swim you'll find tampons better than sanitary towels which will get water-logged.

Sexual Intercourse

As you read this 6,000,000 people in the world are having sex.

You may know all about sex and how to 'do it', but there will be quite a few who will read this book who won't know. So this is for them. You can skip it if you know it all.

Sexual intercourse is a physical act

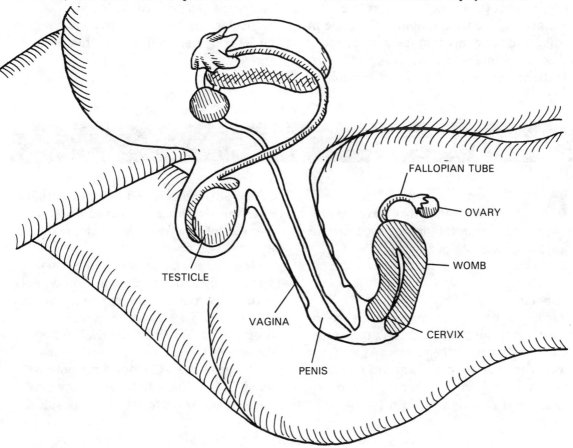

FALLOPIAN TUBE

OVARY

WOMB

TESTICLE

CERVIX

VAGINA

PENIS

whereby a man inserts his penis into the vagina of a woman.

Both partners may be excited about the thought of sex. For the man this is almost essential, because without excitement and stimulation his penis is unlikely to become stiff and rigid. Then it will be hard − if that is the right word − for the penis to be placed inside the woman. This erection happens as blood fills up spongy tissue within the penis. As the woman gets excited the vagina becomes wet and more receptive to her partner.

Female orgasm, or orgasms, may occur at any stage of sexual intercourse. The climax of intercourse for the man is the ejaculation (often called 'coming') of about four millilitres of semen. This is squirted out from the penis into the deepest part of the vagina − the site of the neck of the womb. Some of the sperm will make their way into the womb, and then along one of the two fallopian tubes. If they meet an ovum then fertilization may take place. After fertilization the egg travels down into the womb and may implant in its wall. This is the start of nine months of growth within the womb. At the end of that time, if all has gone according to plan, a new being − a baby − is born into the world down the vagina.

As you might expect from an act that can produce a baby, and which involves such close contact and pleasure, the emotions concerned with sex are not just physical. Many people believe sex should be reserved for marriage, or at least a stable relationship. Sex involves love and respect and caring for a person. Having sex with casual partners brings an increased risk of disease, and for women an increased risk of cancer of the neck of the womb. The risk of AIDS, in particular, has made the 'free love' notion far less popular than it was a few years ago.

Contraception

Most couples do not wish to have a baby every time they have sex, and so the human race has devised various ways of preventing pregnancy. These are called methods of contraception.

Condom

Barrier method. The man wears a rubber sheath over the erect penis, and this stops the sperm entering the vagina. As well as condoms these get called various names such as French letter, johnnys, or rubber johnnys. It is fairly reliable if put on before any contact, and removed carefully afterwards without any semen being allowed into the vagina. Condoms should only be used once.

Advantages. Condoms can be bought fairly easily and cheaply, and you do not need to see a doctor to get them. They are easy to use. They also give good protection against sexually transmitted diseases (STDs).

Disadvantages. Condoms are not one hundred per cent safe because they may burst, leak, or come off. Some people do

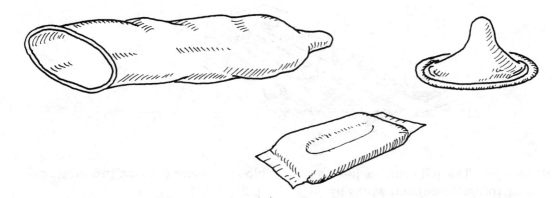

not like using them. They feel there is some loss of sensation. It is very important that they are rolled onto the erect penis before any sexual contact.

Cap or diaphragm

This is a barrier method used by women. Some form of cap covers the neck of the womb, so that sperm cannot get by to the egg. It is put in before sex takes place. A cap or diaphragm must be used with spermicides which inactivate sperm. It is reliable if used correctly.

Advantages. There is no loss of sensation. It does not affect the female hormones and it gives some protection against STDs.

Disadvantages. You have to remember to fit a cap or diaphragm before sex. This is fairly easy but needs to be learnt from a doctor or family planning nurse.

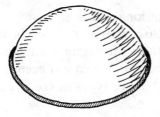

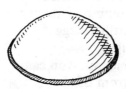

There may be creams (spermicides) also put in the vagina which can act against the sperm. They should be used *with* one of the barrier methods above, and are *not* reliable on their own.

The contraceptive pill

Oral contraceptive, the birth pill or just 'the pill.' This is one of the most reliable methods of contraception. It is taken regularly by the woman, and stops the egg being released from the ovary. It contains two hormones – an oestrogen and a progestogen.

Advantages. It is almost one hundred per cent reliable and it does not interfere with sexual intercourse.

Disadvantages. It interferes with the body's own hormones. It can only be given by a doctor. There is no protection from STD.

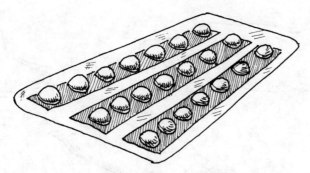

The mini-pill. This pill contains just one hormone (progestogen) and works by making if difficult for the sperm to get by the cervix.

Advantages. There is less risk of raised blood pressure than the two-hormone 'pill'.

Disadvantages. It is not so reliable as the 'pill' and it has to be taken exactly the same time each day.

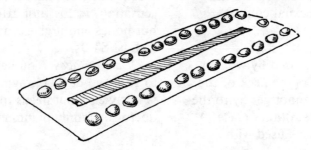

The coil A coil (or IUD − intrauterine device) is placed in the womb by a doctor and will usually stop a fertilized egg implanting and developing.

Advantages. It is reliable, and you can forget all about it apart from the occasional check-up.

Disadvantages. A coil is not usually suitable for young women as it may cause infection. It also has been known to fall out! Three types of coil are shown here.

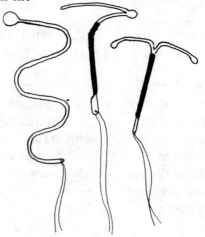

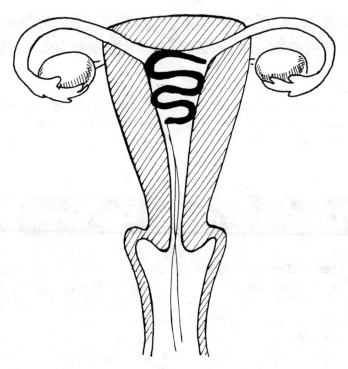

The rhythm method

The rhythm method of contraception involves predicting the time of the month when an egg is released and avoiding intercourse around that time.

Advantages. There aren't many apart from the lack of preparation.

Disadvantages. It isn't always easy to get the timing of this method right and if you get it wrong there is no other contraceptive method used to prevent egg fertilization.

Coitus interruptus.

This relies on the withdrawal of the penis before ejaculation.

Advantages. Like the rhythm method, there aren't many apart from the lack of preparation.

Disadvantages. It isn't very satisfying physically. It is also very unreliable as sperm may enter the woman's vagina during intercourse before the man ejaculates.

Saying 'no'

Either boy or girl can use this method.

Advantages. There is no way the girl can get pregnant. No STDs. And many more.

Disadvantages. None.

Keeping your fingers crossed is not a form of contraception.

Morning after pill. If a girl has unprotected sex there is a 'morning after pill' available from your doctor or family planning clinic. Act fast if you need this help — at least within seventy-two hours (three days) of having sex without any precautions.

Sexual Intercourse and the Law

In the UK it is still illegal for a male to have sexual intercourse with a female below the age of sixteen − the age of consent. While the law may turn a 'blind eye' to such activity, this is not always so. In particular, when the male is over eighteen years of age prosecution may follow unlawful sexual intercourse.

Sexually Transmitted Disease [STD]

There are a number of diseases which can be passed between partners during sex. Not all of them are serious, and most can be treated fairly easily. The quicker treatment begins the better.

AIDS

AIDS is a disease which can be caught in several ways, but for most people the only real risk comes from having sexual intercourse with an infected person.

The letters AIDS stand for Acquired Immune Deficiency Syndrome. The disease is caused by the Human Immunodeficiency Virus, which is usually known as HIV.

The virus attacks the body's natural immune defences. Without an immune system, as was mentioned earlier, the body is wide open to infections and some cancers.

You may not know that you have AIDS for up to eight years after you acquire the virus. During this time you are infectious and can pass it on. A blood test can detect if a person is HIV positive or negative. When AIDS develops the patient feels generally awful. He or she loses weight and glands in the body go lumpy.

At the moment there is no cure or vaccine against AIDS. People with the disease become ill and die from illnesses they cannot fight off.

You catch AIDS by getting body fluids (principally semen, vaginal fluid and blood) into your body. This may happen if you have any form of unprotected sex with an infected person − the act of anal sex seems to be the riskiest. The infected person may look perfectly well; many people carry the virus without any sign of ill health.

Using a condom correctly during sex will give some protection against AIDS, although this is not one hundred per cent safe as condoms may split or come off.

Sharing needles, syringes and other equipment connected with drug misuse is also likely to result in AIDS being passed on.

During pregnancy HIV may pass from an infected mother to her baby.

It is actually quite difficult to catch AIDS. The virus is not passed on by everyday activities like sharing rooms, sneezing, coughing or shaking hands with an infected person.

Venereal disease

There is often confusion about terms used for these conditions. Many adults, for example, consider the term VD means all disease caught from sexual contact. This is not correct.

Venereal Disease (VD) is a term not used much these days. VD is legally defined as either syphilis, gonorrhoea, or an infection called chancroid. These are all quite uncommon nowadays in the UK and they are always passed from one person to another by sexual activity.

On the other hand sexually transmitted diseases (STDs) are most often contracted during a sexual act, but need *not* necessarily be picked up in this way. Put simply this means that if you need to go to an STD clinic it does not mean that you have caught VD.

Syphilis
Syphilis, or 'the pox' as it was once known, is caused by an organism called a spirochaete. The first sign of the disease for anyone who has syphilis is a painless sore on the body. This is usually where sexual contact has taken place. So it usually appears on the penis or vagina.

Antibiotics are used to treat syphilis, though the disease is rare these days. If it is left untreated for years, as sometimes happened in days gone by, brain damage can result.

Gonorrhoea
Gonorrhoea is also known as 'the clap' and it is caused by a bacteria. Men with gonorrhoea show a yellow discharge from the penis and passing urine can be painful, with a feeling like passing fragments of glass. Women suffering from gonorrhoea usually notice nothing, though there may be a vaginal discharge, a lower belly ache, or pain on passing water.

Once diagnosed, gonorrhea is usually very easy to cure with antibiotics.

NSU (Non-specific urethritis)
This is an infection of the urethra in males, for which it is often impossible to pinpoint a cause. It hurts males with NSU to pass water and they may feel the need to go more frequently. There may also be discharge from the penis.

Women do not get symptoms of NSU as the germs which cause it rarely live and cause symptoms in the female urethra.

However, these germs can be found in abundance in the vagina and around the cervix and this is how they are passed to the male.

NSU may follow intercourse with a regular partner, and may indicate that the vagina has an infection (like thrush which is described shortly) that can be acquired non-sexually. So it is possible to get an NSU even if both partners are faithful to one another.

Wearing a condom will prevent NSU.

Antibiotics will usually clear up NSU.

Genital warts
These are caused by a virus and appear as fleshy warts on the genitals. Special paint to treat them is available from a doctor.

There may be a link between genital

warts and cancer of the cervix. So women who have had such warts should have regular smear tests.

Pubic lice

Pubic lice, or 'crabs', are small lice which cause itching around the genitals and in pubic hair. You can see them if you look carefully. Again a special lotion is available to get rid of them. And, as with all STDs, the person who you caught the lice from must get treatment or you may get them back.

Genital herpes

This is caused by the herpes virus and appears as painful sores around the penis and vagina. There is no real cure for genital herpes but a doctor can give something to bring some relief.

Blisters will disappear but they may recur from time to time.

Trichomonas (TV)

A microbe called trichomonas vaginalis is the cause of this, hence the name TV. The disease causes a vaginal irritation and smelly, often green, discharge. It is treated by the drug metronidazole (Flagyl) taken by mouth.

TV may infect the male without giving symptoms and both partners usually need treatment.

Another infection which is sometimes sexually transmitted is thrush. However, thrush is quite common among people who have never had sex.

Thrush is caused by a yeast called

candida and the infection causes a red itchy penis or a white, creamy vaginal discharge.

Anti-yeast cream from a doctor, often combined with a vaginal pessary of the same anti-yeast medicine for the female is used to treat thrush.

There are other infections that people can get from sexual contact. However it is important to know that sex is a normal, healthy and very pleasant part of life. There are ways to avoid STDs and so do not let this list of diseases make sex appear dirty or dangerous.

Sensible precautions to avoid catching STD

1. By being faithful to one person. Otherwise limiting the number of partners. The more people you have sex with the more chance of a STD.
2. Barrier methods, e.g. a condom, help prevent the spread of STDs.
3. Do not have sex if you are unsure about your own or your partner's health, as regards STDs. Anyone who thinks he or she may have such a problem should seek medical help.

Remember it is very possible to be infected with one of these diseases and not to know it.

Clinics

These are now called GU Medicine clinics. (GU stands for Genito-Urinary.) They used to be called VD clinics, and subsequently Special Treatment Clinics. Every major town has at least one clinic. Treatment and advice given in these clinics is free, and the advice is confidential. No-one will be told that you have gone to one if you do not wish.

The address of your nearest clinic may be found in the telephone directory or on notices displayed in main public toilets. This information is often found in the toilets of discos and night clubs.

If in any doubt simply ring the switchboard of the nearest large hospital and you will either be put through to a clinic or given the necessary information.

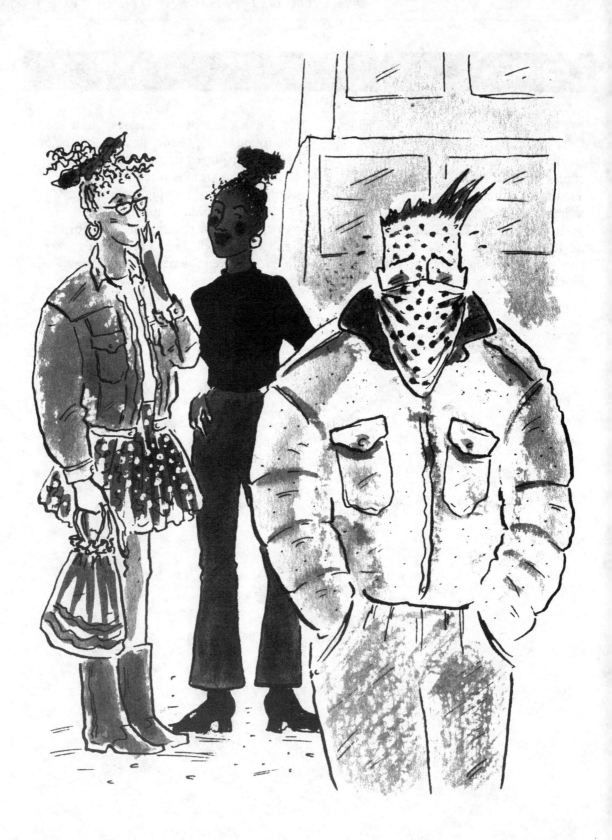

3

Well, Well . . . Well?

Acne

Spots can be a real nuisance when you are a teenager, and they often seem to appear when you want to look your best. First the facts about spots, and then how to best deal with them. Read on if you have spots because help is at hand.

Acne affects about eight in ten teenagers. It is certainly the commonest skin problem affecting young people. Some get these spots worse than others. As far as I know nobody has ever died of acne, but it may be a dreadful, disfiguring, miserable condition.

The underlying cause is the change in body hormones which are taking place in the teens. The level of these hormones increases, and one effect of this is to make glands in the skin (sebaceous glands − see page 13) produce an excess of the oily substance (sebum) that keeps skin soft and healthy. This oil clogs up the openings of these glands to produce a plug of partially dried grease. These are known as blackheads, and they cause a

further build up of sebum which can get infected and may cause large boils to form. The condition is so common it hardly needs any further description.

The areas of the body usually affected are the face, neck and chest, because these are where the grease glands are commonest. For obvious reasons people with a tendency to a greasy skin usually suffer more. In girls, periods − because of hormone changes − may make spots worse. Everyone will tell you that you'll grow out of spots. It's true − usually by the age of twenty-five at the latest − however if you are twelve that's over a whole lifetime away!

Although acne cannot be prevented, there is a *lot* you can do to stop scarring, and to make the problem bearable.

You must be prepared to help yourself. If you're not worried by spots − fine. But if you want to get rid of them, then some effort is needed.

DIY Spot Fighting Guide

1. Keep your skin clean. This means washing it twice a day with medicated (antiseptic soap) and carefully drying it afterwards.
2. Avoid getting the skin greasy. Some foundation creams, for example, will make acne worse.
3. Sunlight will tend to make acne better. This does not mean getting sunburnt – a bad move at any time.
4. You can buy treatments from the chemist to put on the skin. Experiment with these and find the one that suits you. The most expensive are not necessarily the best. Some are available from the doctor, and if you are under sixteen you will not have to pay. It is important with many of these treatments to continue for at least two months. You cannot expect instant results with the antibiotics your doctor may give you for example. So don't get disheartened and stop the treatment if there isn't an immediate improvement.
5. Try not to make a habit of squeezing spots. If you must squeeze one wash your hands and clean under your nails first.
6. Go to the doctor for help if you can not control acne yourself. There are many modern and very effective treatments. Some antibiotics which you will need to swallow will help as many as seventy per cent of patients with spots.

TOP FIVE MYTHS ABOUT ACNE

1. Having sex and masturbating will not make spots worse.
2. Chocolates, spicy food and greasy food will not cause spots.
3. The black in blackheads is a pigment *not* dirt.
4. Acne is not catching.
5. Spots are not a sign of disease. They are just a part of growing up.

Warts

These harmless lumpy skin growths are caused by the human wart virus. They often appear in groups on the body. They are spread by direct contact with an infected person. If they occur on the soles of the feet, the weight of the body flattens them. These warts are often called verruca which means 'wart' in Latin.

Warts often disappear of their own accord, but sometimes preparations bought at the chemists or obtained from a doctor can be applied to help them on their way.

Alcohol.

Alcohol is a drug. It just happens to be one that is not illegal once you are a certain age. If you intend to drink alcohol you must know what a dangerous drug it can be. Just because it is legal doesn't take away any of the problems that come with drinking to excess.

Getting drunk — even on a single occasion — may result in violence, personal injury (bar fights), road traffic accidents, accidents in the home, and drownings.

Prolonged drinking over a number of years may produce dependence on alcohol. This is a fairly slow process and it is very easy to slip quietly into the state without realizing it. Complete recovery is possible, but it is far better to treat alcohol with respect and not end up in this condition. Most people know that excess alcohol can damage the liver. However prolonged excess drinking may also damage other organs such as the brain and the heart.

Caffeine

You may not think of caffeine, which is found in some popular drinks like tea and coffee, as a drug but it has a number of complex effects. It works by stimulating the brain and nervous system. It speeds up thought processes and delays both mental and physical fatigue. The dose of caffeine necessary to do this varies between 100–300mg. In large doses of over 1000mg there are a number of unpleasant side effects including restlessness, fast heart rate (palpitations), trembling and

difficulty sleeping. This table gives an idea of the amount of caffeine in popular drinks. These are only average figures; if you drink strong coffee, for example, you will have a higher dose of caffeine than you do drinking weak coffee. Remember too that some of these can be bought 'decaffeinated'.

Cup of coffee 100–200mg
Cup of tea   50–100mg
Cup of cocoa 50–200mg
Bottle of cola 35–50mg

Tobacco

It may well be that you have decided that you might start to smoke cigarettes. Perhaps you already have. Anyway as this is basically a free country, if you decide you wish to smoke, you'll

probably succeed one way or another. However there are some facts you should know about what you are taking on.

The first is that it is unlikely that you will live as long a life if you smoke. The average smoker of twenty-five cigarettes a day will lose about five years of life. Another way of looking at it is that forty per cent of smokers die before they retire from work — this compares with fifteen per cent of non-smokers. These statistics can be juggled around in various ways. Here's another. The age of thirty-five may seem a long way off but . . .

Percentage of men of thirty-five who may expect to die before the age of sixty-five.

1. Non-smokers   15%
2. Smokers   (1 – 14 cigs/day)   22%
3. Smokers   (15 – 24 cigs/day)   25%
4. Smokers (more than 25 cigs/day) 40%

This doesn't mean you are certain to die young. Some lucky smokers live a long life. Just as some people sometimes win on fruit machines in amusement arcades. (Although I've never heard of anyone making a regular living out of it.)

So if you have started smoking you may be interested to know why you began. Research shows that you will begin because you wanted to look 'tough' or 'grown-up'. Research also reveals that by the age of twenty, people are largely divided into either smokers or non-smokers. After that age you continue to smoke for different reasons. The most powerful one is that you are addicted to the drug nicotine in tobacco. This drug nicotine can make it very very difficult to stop.

There are three main diseases caused by smoking.

1. Heart disease is dramatically increased in smokers. Nicotine makes the heart beat faster, and with an increased blood pressure, the heart has to work harder. As well as the increased pressure there is less oxygen in the blood. So you will have about double the chance of suffering a heart attack.

The circulation of the blood is affected in another way. Tobacco smoking causes blood vessels to fur up and become narrowed. The result is that less blood is able to get through these vessels, and vital organs such as the brain and the kidneys may become damaged.

2. Cancer of the lung is often the end result of smoking. Nine out of ten people with this cancer are smokers or ex-smokers.

3. Smoking slowly destroys the lungs — even without the help of cancer. Over the years this gets worse. Eventually when non-smokers are enjoying an active retirement, many smokers have so much trouble breathing that they can't walk.

There are other diseases caused by smoking — poor circulation of the blood to the legs may cause gangrene — but the above three are the really common ones. Some people do manage to stop smoking and there are substantial advantages to this. You will have a lot more money to spend on other things. You will taste and smell better. Also, as soon as you stop smoking your risk of dying young starts to recede, and eventually approaches that of someone who has never smoked.

And finally, you ought to know if you are going to start smoking, that each year in this country smoking kills over 100,000 people. That's about the same as a jumbo jet crashing *every day* and killing all its passengers. Are you sure you wish to be on that flight?

Drugs

Unless you lead a very sheltered life it is quite possible that as a teenager you will be offered some form of illegal drug. Sometimes drugs are offered as a mixture, such as heroin and cocaine.

Main dangers of drugs

1. Overdose. Heroin, for example, can easily produce unconsciousness. It is very difficult to get the dose 'right' with these drugs since they are often mixed ('cut') with other substances.
2. Accidents can easily follow drug taking for obvious reasons.
3. Dependency may follow regular use as many of these drugs 'hook' you.
    Also many produce what is called tolerance. This comes with repeated use, and means more of the drug needs to be taken to produce the same effect.

Marijuana

1. This drug is basically a plant. It comes in many forms and has many names: Cannabis, blow, pot, dope, grass, and ganja.
2. Marijuana is usually smoked in a pipe or as a cigarette.
3. Accidents mainly happen while under the influence of marijuana. Also it is likely to bring users into contact with more dangerous drugs. Long-term use affects memory, impairs sexual performance, and learning ability.

Amphetamines

1. Speed, uppers, whizzers. Usually come as tablets.
2. Taken in tablet form and also sniffed and injected. It stimulates the nervous system – hence its slang names.
3. After the giggly 'high' phase, users often become depressed and have difficulty sleeping. Heavy use brings a feeling of being persecuted.

Ecstasy

1. 'E', XTC, Adam, white doves, disco-burgers, Dennis the Menaces. Usually comes as white tablets,
2. Taken by mouth. Brings a sensation of well-being and alertness.
3. After use, follows a feeling of depression and creeping anxiety.

Cocaine

1. Coke, and in one form 'crack'. This drug comes as a white powder.
2. It is usually sniffed but can be smoked and injected.
3. The effects are similar to amphetamines. Users become dependent ('hooked') on cocaine and it can be very difficult to stop.

Heroin

1. H, smack, skag, and gear. This drug usually comes as a powder.
2. It can be injected, smoked or sniffed.

3. A very addictive drug with very unpleasant withdrawal symptoms.

Glue and other inhaled solvents

1. Comes in various packaging.
2. These solvents are usually inhaled.
3. Sometimes sniffing butane (lighter fuel) gas can cause sudden death. The common danger of solvent abuse is having some sort of accident while under the influence. (About one hundred people, mostly teenagers, died in this way in 1990.)

LSD

1. Acid. Sold in various ways. It may be used to lace drinks and is often sold impregnated on paper.
2. LSD is taken by mouth.
3. It produces over-excitement and may cause the user to do something damaging which seems possible while under the drug's influence. For instance, users may believe they can fly and jump out of a window. Also frightening hallucinations and confusion may result.

The risk involved with injecting drugs is very great. They include AIDS, hepatitis, blood poisoning, and abscesses.

Using these drugs and dealing in them is illegal. Penalties are often very severe, especially for selling them or supplying to others. For example simply possessing heroin can lead to seven years in jail.

Penalties abroad are often even more severe. Some countries have the death sentence if you are caught with these drugs.

However if you have a problem with them you can go for help to a doctor or an agency which specializes in drug problems. There is no fear of prosecution if you ask for this help.

Glandular Fever

This illness is caused by a virus. So it's passed on by contact with someone who has got glandular fever. There are many jokes made about it for two reasons:

1. It is hardly ever fatal. So because you will not die of it people may not take it too seriously.
2. It is also called the 'kissing disease'.

Glandular fever (also called infectious mononucleosis) is spread from one person to another by intimate contact such as kissing. The main symptoms are a sore throat, tiredness, and generalized aches and pains.

The main signs are enlargement of the lymph glands — the body's own natural defences against infection. Although serious complications are unusual, the symptom of tiredness may drag on for several months. There is no cure for this.

So a long boring convalescence at home may be needed. You can arrange for some school work to be sent home, and you may want to do a little if you feel up to it.

The Common Cold

This is a viral infection which effects the lining in the nose and throat. It lasts about a week and there is no cure yet. Very many different viruses cause 'colds' and they are changing all the time. This means that making a vaccine against 'colds' is not practical.

The ten most 'popular' symptoms of a cold (100 young adults were asked)

1.	Runny nose	100%
2.	Blocked nose	99%
3.	Sneezing	97%
4.	Sore or dry throat	96%
5.	'Unwell'	81%
6.	Discharge down back of throat	79%
7.	Headache	78%
8.	Cough	76%
9.	Feeling hot	49%
10.	Burning eyes	28%

(Muscle aching fails to make the charts with only 22% of the vote.)

Colds are not caught by being cold and wet. If they were it seems unlikely that anyone could climb Mount Everest without a load of tissues the size of the mountain itself. Feeling cold is often the first sign of a cold so it is easy to blame 'feeling cold' for the infection.

They are commoner in winter when it happens to be cold because:

1. Winter happens to be the time of the year when the cold viruses are most active.
2. People crowd together in schools and offices with the windows shut and pass the virus on very efficiently.

Treatment. There is no cure, but symptoms can be helped by keeping warm and taking small doses of paracetamol medicine regularly. Antibiotics will not help an uncomplicated 'cold'.

Body Odour – Being Smelly

Of the five senses (the others are touch, sight, hearing and taste) smell is the one which is most easily 'forgotten'. This is handy if you work in a sewer because after the first few minutes the unpleasant smell does not register anymore. (It works the other way around too with perfume.) It does mean that you are unlikely to smell yourself if you have body odour or BO.

Other people will smell it very quickly though when they meet you. And it only takes a second to go off someone. So if you meet someone you fancy, you are unlikely to get on if their first deep breath of you hits them like a smelly sock with a brick in it.

Sweat does not smell. What does smell is sweat which has been left on the body for some time. Sweat evaporates very quickly from many parts of the body — the face for example. However in nooks and crannies like the armpits, feet (with shoes and socks on) and of course the genitalia which are usually covered by clothes, skin bacteria have time to break the sweat down into substances that do smell. This doesn't happen that quickly so if you wash regularly and use a deodorant, if necessary, there should be no problem.

Some people sweat more than others but that really isn't an excuse. No-one should have body odour unless they want to.

Athletes' Foot

This is a common skin infection of the feet caused by a fungus. Swimming pools and showers are the places to pick this up because the fungus likes the warm wet atmosphere found in them. If you have sweaty feet and wear nylon socks that do not absorb sweat like cotton, so much the better as far as the fungus is concerned. Cover the lot with shoes and the fungus is ecstatic!

Smelly, itchy feet with white skin beneath and between the toes are what you will probably notice. If the fungus gets into the toe nails they become thick and yellow.

You can avoid the problem by washing your feet every day, and putting on clean cotton socks. Change your footwear fairly often so — trainers especially — they have time to dry out.

Athletes' foot is not serious, but tackle it quickly and it's easy to get rid of. If these measures do not work, the doctor will supply some cream or powder and this should work quickly as long as you stick to the basic foot hygiene outlined above. It is important to continue using cream for at least two weeks after infection appears to have cleared. This greatly reduces the chance of a relapse.

If the fungus gets into the nails then you may be prescribed some tablets. They usually have to be taken for as long as six to nine months for finger nails, and one year to eighteen months for toe nails.

Allergy

This is an over-reaction by the body to some substance or substances. There are two main types of allergy — immediate and delayed.

Immediate allergy may cause nettle rashes, hay fever, and asthma. Common causes of this type of allergy are: pollen, house dust, strawberries and shellfish. Of course there are hundreds more, many of which go undiscovered.

Delayed allergy may occur with many substances including cheap metals (causing dermatitis), perfume, and sticking plaster.

Conditions in which allergies are important:

Hay fever.
Asthma.
Some types of eczema.

Hay fever

Hay fever is a common reaction to grass pollens in summer. Common symptoms are a blocked runny nose and itchy, watery eyes. It is worth remembering that such symptoms can occur at any time. It depends on what you are allergic to. So if you are allergic to the house dust mite you may notice these symptoms of allergy when you make your bed. The mite likes the warm and slight damp of bedding. If your nose runs only on Saturday morning when you help at the local riding school then you may be allergic to something around horses and their stables.

General advice

1. Avoid grassy areas if possible, and stay inside when the lawn is being mown.
2. Keep car and house windows shut as much as possible during the season. Sun glasses may help.
3. Make your school aware of your difficulty — especially at exam times. They can often make allowances for the problem and may be able to help.
4. If possible try and get away to the seaside at half-term and weekends during the hay fever season as sea breezes tend to be free of pollen.

There are a lot of medicines now available which can help hay fever sufferers. Some are preventative and need to be taken during the entire hay fever season. Others, like the antihistamines, dampen down the symptoms. Modern antihistamines should not make you sleepy.

Asthma

Asthma is a transient and reversible narrowing of the airways in the lungs. You may notice anything from a dry cough to audible wheezing. There are many other symptoms too such as coughing up plugs of white phlegm, a tight chest and difficulty in breathing.

If bacteria invade the narrowed airways then bronchitis results, and you may notice the phlegm turns yellow or green.

Like the treatment for hay fever, some treatments relieve the symptoms and others attempt to prevent attacks. Inhalers are favourite ways of delivering the drugs because these devices place the medicine right where it's needed — in the lungs. If an infection complicates an asthma attack you may need to take a course of antibiotics.

Eczema

Eczema is also known as dermatitis. It is a type of inflammation of the skin. There are a variety of forms of the problem and they may be related to an allergy.

Treatment aims to reduce the symptoms by softening the skin and reducing the itching. The skin should be kept clean and soft. There are a number of creams and oils which will prevent the skin from drying out. Steroid creams can produce a dramatic, if temporary, improvement to eczema. Use them as instructed.

As well as medicine, the itchy skin often benefits from cotton clothes. Wool and nylon frequently make the irritation worse.

Motion Sickness

This happens when the body's balance mechanism is upset by movement. There are a series of spirit levels in the inner ear. These work together with the eyes to keep the body well balanced. If the brain gets confusing messages from these two sources of information then sickness may be the result.

Other factors may add to the problem. An early morning cross-Channel trip with last night's double hamburger, chips and beans still in the stomach is asking for trouble. Also if you expect to be sick then there is a better chance that you will be. It can happen in trains and boats and planes as well as on such things as fair ground rides.

Travel sickness is better prevented than cured. (It is often said that the only certain way to avoid the problem is to sit under an oak tree!)

1. Do not travel on a full stomach if you suffer with this problem. However do have a light snack before you go.

2. There are several medicines that you can buy over the counter. Tell your pharmacist − or doctor − how long the journey will be. There are many very effective medicines and they act for different lengths of time. You will not want a short acting one if you are flying to Australia. On the other hand you do not want one that acts for a day if it is not necessary. Some of these medicines may make you a bit sleepy.

At the risk of stating the obvious you must take the medicines before the journey. It is unhelpful to wait until you are being sick before you attempt to swallow something.

3. Have a fresh, cool, non-fizzy drink to hand during the journey. Sip this if nausea begins, and it will help it to go away.

Eating Problems

We are fortunately all different shapes and sizes. It would be very boring if we all looked the same. So with a healthy appetite and a good amount of exercise our bodies will stay in the form that was inherited at conception.

However there is a lot of pressure, particularly on teenage girls, to be a 'fashionable' shape. The current 'fashion' is to be thin. (It hasn't always been so. At one time the ideal shape for women was much plumper.)

The desire to be thin and to diet can very easily become an illness. This problem is called anorexia nervosa, and sufferers may be extremely thin and yet still have the idea firmly in mind that their bodies are overweight. It is quite possible to die if you get into this state, and sadly some young people do. Both boys and girls too can suffer with this terrible problem.

Sometimes a patient with an eating disorder may binge on food, and then make themselves physically sick in order to get rid of the food. (This is called bulimia.)

If you think you might be developing such an unhealthy interest in being thin, please go and see someone for help quickly. If you haven't got this problem, well it doesn't matter that you have checked it out. However, it is a very dangerous illness to ignore.

Eating problems are interwoven with stress, depression and anxiety, which follow in the next chapter.

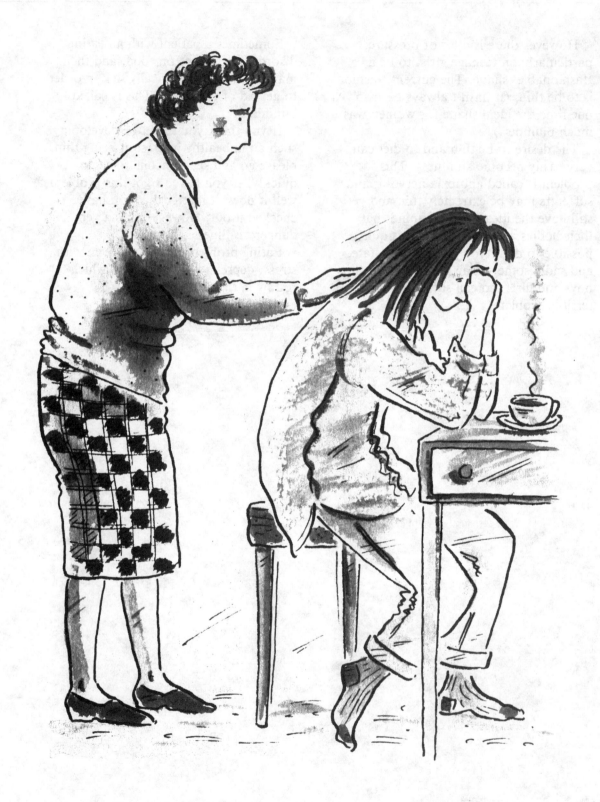

4

Down in the Dumps

At one time we all led lives where we lived in caves and hunted animals for food. We chased them, and some of them chased us. If you didn't catch your food you went hungry. If you got caught yourself you might die. The outcome of a fight over the best cave or a fancied mate would literally be a life and death matter.

All this was powered by body hormones like adrenalin. This substance pours out of glands above the kidneys and gets you ready to run or fight. It speeds up the heart, increases breathing, and sends blood to where it will be needed. So the muscles get more at the expense of the areas like the skin, which can be seen to go white.

All this is fine if you really do need a fast heart rate and more oxygen in the lungs. But things have changed from the days of living in caves. We still have fights over the same things – like where to live, partners and work – but these days they are done from behind school desks, at interviews and on the phone. There is usually no need to use the energy to actually run and fight. However, the

adrenalin pours out all the same – and that may produce the signs and symptoms of stress.

Remember that stress is a normal part of life that we all have to face. It is not necessarily bad. Things would be very unexciting without it. It is how your body deals with it that is important.

If you handle stress badly, then there are not only mental problems but physical signs that can be seen and measured. These problems are never 'all in the mind'. Mind and body go together.

Physical feelings

- Fast 'thumping' heart. Often called palpitations.
- Sweating – mainly under the arms and palms of hands.
- Running to the loo. (Either diarrhoea or urge to pass water.)
- Not able to sleep as well as usual.
- Feeling dizzy.
- Headaches. Often like a tight band around the head or up the back of the neck spreading onto the top of the head.

- Feeling sick and weak − 'butterflies in stomach'. Legs wobbly. Mouth dry and you feel like swallowing a lot.
- Pins and needles in the hands and feet, and sometimes around the mouth.

Changes in behaviour

Apart from these physical feelings there are changes in a person's behaviour when stress and anxiety are a problem. Other people may notice these in you before you do yourself. It is worth asking your best friend if you suspect something has changed in your behaviour.

Here are a few things that commonly happen.

- Loss of interest in things which would normally be fun, like: sex, going to a disco, holidays. General feeling of can't be bothered. Always too tired.
- Loss of confidence. You begin to worry about simple things which normally would present no problems, such as walking into a classroom and having to meet someone. This naturally brings an increase in the need for reassurance, and you are constantly seeking advice that all is well.
- Mood changes. You become tearful and erratic. One minute you are fine, the next you have lost your temper or break down in tears because of something silly. Instead of your usual easy going laid back way of doing things you are rigid and strict with yourself. Things have to be exact and 'right'. If they are not exactly as you think they should be, you get upset; e.g. someone at home is five minutes

late posting a letter for you and you explode.

Questionnaire − Are you vulnerable to stress? It is important to answer the questions as truthfully as possible. Mark what you *would* do in real life. Not what you think is the best answer.

A_____

One Monday morning you go to school knowing you are going to meet someone who does not like you. This person is very good at bullying and can always think of a good put down line. Over the weekend you have heard from a friend that for some reason you have annoyed this person, and he or she is going to 'get' you. Which of these is most likely to be you on the way to school that morning.

1. Arm yourself with something like a half brick.
2. Talk about the problem with your best friend.
3. Say nothing and think hard about what could happen.
4. Stay at home and say you feel sick.

Discussion. This sort of worry is best handled by talking about it (2). Certainly not by violence (1). Dodging the issue (4) only puts off the problem. And worrying alone (3) won't help either.

B_____

You have become involved with the police, and face a court appearance over some vandalism at school. Graffiti was sprayed on some walls. You didn't actually handle the paint, but were present when the police arrived.

Which of these statements most closely fits how you think you would feel.

1. Rather proud to be involved in this adventure.

2. Have lied to the police — and are not worried as you feel able to explain to the court that it was nothing to do with you.
3. Have talked to your parents about the problem. They are coming to court with you.
4. The incident has caused a massive row with the people who were caught with you. Once all friends, everyone is now blaming one another.

Discussion. Talking over these sorts of scrapes (3) is a great help. Not only will your parents be likely to help you in practical ways, but knowing they will stand by you is very reassuring. Falling out with 'friends' (4) brings unnecessary stress. A court appearance for any offence is always stressful unless you are a complete idiot (1). Lying to the police and the court could land you in even deeper trouble (2).

C_____

One of your family is killed in a car crash. You feel very unhappy. Do you:

1. Refuse to discuss the matter as it makes you cry and get upset. For the same reason you refuse to go to the funeral.
2. Your family doctor has a nurse attached to the practice. You make an appointment to see her.
3. Have a few drinks whenever you feel sad.
4. Get involved with something illegal such as shoplifting which seems to take your mind off things.

Discussion. Grief is a natural emotion, which should not be suppressed (1). It would be unnatural not to feel sad if someone close to you died — especially in tragic circumstances. Alcohol (3) is only a short-term answer and brings problems of its own. So does any sort of illegal activity (4). Your family doctor and the practice nurse are both skilled in ways of helping in these circumstances. Ways of discussing the situation — often called counselling (2) — will sort this out.

D_____

You have moved bedroom to the front of the house for a month or so while granny stays in your bedroom. There is more traffic noise at night, and you are not sleeping so well. Do you:

1. Take a small glass of sherry on the quiet at bed time.
2. Ring a double glazing salesman without your parents' knowledge.
3. Take some exercise before going to bed.
4. Refuse to stay in that bedroom and attempt to move back to your previous one.

Discussion. Family rows are stressful. It is not a good idea to force your way back towards granny's temporary room (4); or to call in a double glazing salesman who will arrive and not take 'no' for an answer (2)!

Exercise (3) is a good antidote for this temporary period of stress and will help you to sleep. As for alcohol and surreptitious relief drinking (1) — see answer to C.

E_____

You have been smoking cigarettes for some months when your parents find out. This causes a huge row. What is the nearest to how you would react.

1. Stop smoking and say no more about the matter.

2. Carry on smoking.
3. Say that you are not going to give up and carry on whenever you are able.
4. Visit your family doctor to discuss your next move.

Discussion. Smoking (2) is bad for your health. There is no doubt about that. Lying to your parents (3) and being caught smoking again will cause an even bigger row. Once you become addicted to the nicotine it may be quite stressful to stop without some support (1) and advice from an expert such as the family doctor. Give up with some professional advice (4).

That part of the test measures how vulnerable to stress you are. Some people love pressure, and do well under it. Others crumble. However we all face it every day.

You might like to see how much stress there is in your life at the moment. Mark which of these have happened to you — from the causes of greatest stress (the first group) to the causes of least severe stress (but stress all the same) in the last group.

Death of a parent, or brother, or sister.
Break up of your family. (Parents divorce.)
In trouble with police, with court appearance.
Bad illness or accident. (Knocked over by car and break leg, or involved with unwanted pregnancy.)

Friend dies.
New brother or sister.

Change school.
Move house. (New area.)
Important exams.
New job, or lose a job.
Short of money.

Do something unusually good. (Win a TV quiz show.)
A parent changes job.
Row over staying out late or getting drunk.
Increase in arguments at home.
Trouble with a particular teacher or relative.
Move house. (Same area.)
Change daily routine in some way (for example become vegetarian).
Brother or sister leaves home or gets married.
Death of a favourite pet.
Owe some money and unable to pay.

Move bedroom.
Christmas.
Holidays.
Change in sleeping pattern, like going to bed late or being woken by traffic.
Staying at someone else's house.
Take up a new hobby (for example join dancing class).
Told off by police for riding bike without lights.
More homework.

What can be done?
You can obviously do a lot to help yourself once you realize what is happening to your body; although it may be necessary to go and see someone like a doctor for more professional help.

The D.I.Y. Approach to Managing Stress

Talk to people about how you feel — parents, a close brother or sister, or a friend. Do this quickly when things go wrong. The problems will mount if you sit brooding over them. So do not bottle feelings up.

With the help of this book realize exactly why you feel as you do, why your hands tingle, or why you feel sick in certain situations at school. The problem becomes much less important when you understand it.

Having understood what is happening you can then learn to either avoid a particular difficulty, or to prepare your body to face it. Try some method of relaxation or meditation. More about these later. There are lots of different ways, and not only do they work but they are not dangerous. Drink and drugs are dangerous if misused.

Some things which are often considered rather boring — like exercise and good regular food — will often help in the battle against stress. Exercise burns up some of the 'energy' of stress, and you will feel better and sleep better. The exercise can be anything you like. Disco dancing is just as good as a muddy cross-country run. Do which you prefer. Another advantage is that exercise often involves meeting people and having new hobbies, such as joining a football club or swimming team.

More Help

Go and see your family doctor for reassurance. One trip may be all that is necessary to let you know that your pounding heart is not a sign that you are having a heart attack. The doctor can help by guiding you in the right direction, and away from false friends such as alcohol. In the short-term there are drugs that can be used, but they are only short-term in the way that a crutch helps someone with a broken leg. No one would dream of walking around with a crutch or stick months after the leg is better.

All this advice is very general. If you have actually decided that you are over-stressed the first thing you want to do is to feel better! Just a slight improvement will encourage you and start things moving in the right direction.

Case History

You do not get on with someone who you see now and again. You are never sure when you will meet them. Every time you think about meeting them you sweat and your hands tingle. It has become more difficult to avoid thinking about meeting them. In fact you lie awake at night going over and over things you will say, and rehearsing arguments in your head. For a week or so you haven't eaten as much as usual, and the muscles at the back of your neck ache at the end of the day.

Plan of Action

There are lots of different ways to relax and so to fight the effects of stress. However there is a safe and simple guide to making a start.

I asked a friend who gets wound up very easily how she unwinds. This is her method. Try it. It is simple and takes less than thirty minutes.

1. I go and lie down in my bedroom. Any room will do as long as it is quiet and I am comfortable. Sometimes I do this in a chair or on the sitting room floor when I am on my own in the house.
2. I close my eyes and think of a rose. You can pick anything you like. It could be a sandy hot holiday beach, a forest glade, or the face of someone you trust and love.
3. I start by tensing up my toes, holding them tense for a few seconds and then relaxing the muscles. Still thinking about my rose and with eyes closed I work my way up through the leg muscles to the rest of the body. Within about five minutes I will be tensing the neck muscles and finally relaxing them.
4. After this I lie quite still and concentrate on breathing. I am still thinking of the rose and my muscles are relaxed. Breathe in through the nose and pause before breathing out slowly through the mouth. It should be a slow breathing exercise, and the breath out should be about twice as long as the breath in.

What my friend has found works for her is, in fact, a mixture of the following techniques. You will come across these names, so this is what they all mean. Start with my friend's method and then go on to learn more about the various ways and find which suits you.

Muscle Relaxation. This is a way of relaxing the muscles of the body. It sounds simple but it can be difficult to know when muscles are in fact tense. If you can learn to control and relax the various muscle groups of the body, like around the neck and shoulders, then mental as well as physical relaxation will follow.

Massage. Massage of the muscles by someone can help in such relaxation.

Sleep. This hardly needs to be described, although it is worth thinking about just what sleep is, because it is so important in fighting stress. Sleep is a state where the eyes are closed, the major postural muscles of the body are relaxed, and the conscious state of mind is suspended. Most of us spend a third of our lives like this and this description shows what an ideal state sleep is to combat stress. Just what all the relaxation and meditation is aiming for.

It is important to realize that normal sleep is healthy, and not the sleep that is created with the help of drink and drugs − or both. You cannot go through life avoiding stress completely. If it is giving you problems and a hard time at the moment then you need to sit down and work out what is happening and why.

Then, either on your own or with help from friends, or medical help either avoid the problem, or if it is unavoidable, control the effects of the stress.

Depression

We all get fed up at some time or another. No normal person feels happy all of the time. However, when does an attack of the 'blues', or feeling cheesed off, actually mean that a person has a depressive illness that needs expert medical attention?

These are some of the feelings that may come with a depression that needs help.

- Feeling guilty about things. You feel you let other people down. You feel worthless.
- Feeling tired a lot so that even minor things are 'too much effort'.
- Loss of interest 'can't be bothered' in things that you would normally find enjoyable − like going out with friends.

- Poor sleeping − especially waking up early in the morning.
- Worrying about your physical health for no reason.
- Unexplained and frequent symptoms such as headache and belly ache.
- Fearful of everyday life. You feel hopeless about things. Loss of weight − a change in eating habits, such as eating less or binge eating and then being sick.
- Crying spells.
- A feeling that you are not physically attractive.
- Avoiding school. Either playing truant, or making excuses to stay at home.

There is, of course, a lot of overlap between depression and anxiety. Any of the 'life events' mentioned on page 48 may be associated with depression.

These feelings or events do not in themselves mean a person is seriously depressed; but if you wonder if you feel more sad than you should, and this feeling continues for more than a few days, or keeps coming back, then it is certainly best to go and ask for medical help.

The symptoms of depression like 'no energy and can't be bothered to do anything' actually make seeking help quite a difficult task. However, do ask for help. You may not realize how ill you are until you get better!

A lot of these symptoms will respond to simple measures such as talking about what problems you feel you may have. Who you go to must depend on who you feel most able to confide in. It may be your parents, a teacher, a friend, a priest, or someone at our local surgery such as the doctor or practice nurse.

Whatever you do, go and talk to someone about this illness if you think you might have become depressed.

A few people who get very depressed feel everyone would be better off without them. They may even begin to think that they would be better off dead. If you have thoughts like this please go and see your doctor as soon as possible.

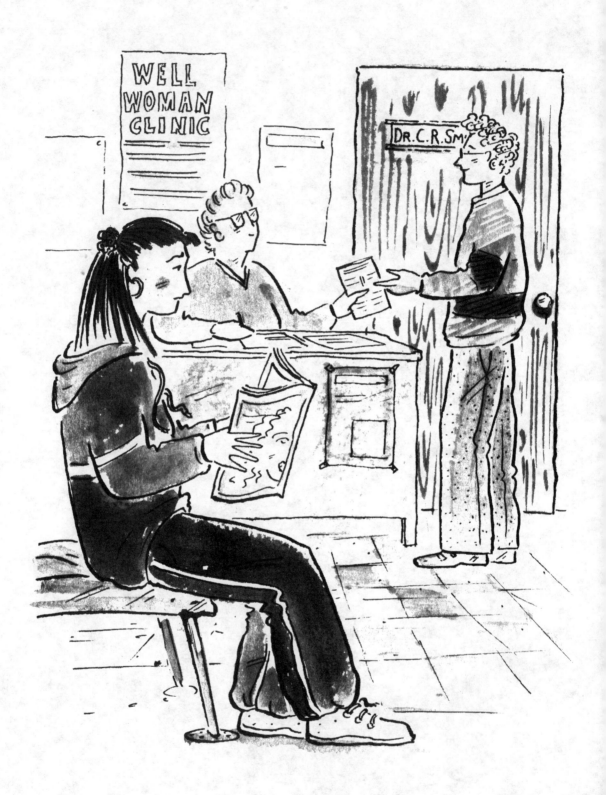

CHAPTER 5

Going to the Doctor

Doctors come in all shapes and sizes! The general practitioner (family doctor) is likely to be the variety you meet at your local surgery. Specialists tend to work in hospitals. Family doctors refer patients with particular problems to these doctors when a very expert opinion about a problem is needed.

So, if you have an itchy rash, the odds are that your local doctor will be able to clear it up. If this is not possible then a doctor who has made rashes and spots his or her whole life's work can be called in.

Family doctor. Family doctors are part of a health team. This team works together to prevent illness as well as to put things right when they go wrong.

Nurse. A practice is likely to have a nurse attached to it. He or she will help the doctor with work such as injections, or dressing wounds. Many nurses are involved in giving routine health checks. This work involves checking − often called screening − healthy people to detect an illness or some other problem early when it can be dealt with easily.

Midwife. A nurse who looks after mothers having babies.

Going to See The Doctor

If you take a look at what doctors do in a busy morning surgery you will get an idea about what the job entails, and what sort of work is done. Every surgery is different − the doctor never knows exactly what problems are going to turn up − but this is fairly typical morning surgery.

Twenty patients seen between 9.00 am and 11.30 am. The average time spent with each patient is about seven minutes. Patients who have made an appointment are booked in every ten minutes. That way they know what time to arrive and do not have to wait long to be seen. Emergencies who can get to the surgery are booked in around these. So everyone who needs to see the doctor that day is attended to.

Some patients need very little time. Perhaps they only need a sick note for work. Others may need longer. Everyone should get the time they need, even if they have to come back later.

As well as seeing ill patients the doctor also gives advice about health, gives vaccinations, and examines healthy people to check that all is well.

At the end of the surgery the doctor will go out and visit patients who need to see a doctor, but who are not able to get to the surgery.

What to Expect from your Doctor

A visit to the doctor usually falls into two parts.

1. You are asked what you feel is wrong.
2. A short examination of you is then done.

Doctors are taught at medical school to examine patients in a precise way so that nothing important is missed. You can pit your wits against our imaginary doctor now as he asks a Miss Rita La Rue to come into his consulting room.

Miss La Rue is a 16-year-old part time disco dancer who has a day job at a local factory which makes ping-pong balls. Her work is to lift up two already pre-glued halves from a conveyor belt, and stick them together to make one complete ping-pong ball. She lives with her Mum and Dad. She has a regular boyfriend – Darren – and has asked to see Dr Elton because she likes him. There is a lady doctor in the practice, but Dr Elton always saw her when she was a child with her earaches, and she likes and trusts him.

'Good morning Miss La Rue. Please sit down.'

'Morning doctor.'

'How can I help you?'

'I've not been myself for about three months doctor.'

'Oh. What was the first thing you noticed?'

'I started to feel a bit sick doctor.'

(The doctor goes on to ask questions and learns that Miss La Rue mainly felt sick in the morning, but that this symptom has now settled. She hasn't had any pain, and hasn't gone off her food. He asks her how much alcohol she drinks since being sick is one sign of excessive drinking. The consultation continues ...)

'You say you haven't had any tummy ache?'

'No doctor. But I often feel bloated, and my stomach sticks out more than it used to. It's difficult to explain really.'

The doctor makes notes about all this in the patient's medical records. He already knows from these where Miss La Rue lives and how old she is. In fact he has been her doctor since she was born. He helped deliver her. He also knows that she works at a local factory where the work can be quite boring. It's also under threat of being closed down.

He goes on to ask her about this and if it's worrying her.'

'No doctor I'm not the worrying kind. Anyway they say I'm the best ball sticker in the place. I'd soon find another job if I lost this one.'

He also asks her if she's been abroad. This is because there are stomach complaints that are rare in the UK but common abroad. It's possible one of these could be behind Rita's symptoms.

Miss La Rue tells the doctor that her last trip abroad was to Spain two years before when she was fourteen. So the Costa Blanca seems an unlikely source of the problem.

She goes on to tell the doctor that she is eating well, has had normal bowel actions and hasn't lost any weight. In fact she thinks she has put some on.

The doctor guides her by asking relevant questions. Some of them do not make much sense to her — she wonders why he wants to know about her holiday in Spain. Still he's a nice man so she tells him anyway.

'Right Miss La Rue, I'd like to examine you. Would you like to go behind the screen and undress as far as your bra and pants. Just cover yourself up with a blanket and I'll be with you in a moment.'

While Rita is undressing, the doctor goes over the problem in his mind. He considers all the common reasons why a young lady like this should have at first felt sick and now feels 'bloated'.

(At this stage you might like to list three reasons why Rita feels like this. Also there is one question that the doctor has not asked that he should have.)

The doctor goes behind the curtains.

'May I lift up the blanket?'

Miss La Rue nods.

The doctor has chosen to examine the abdomen (the part of the body containing the stomach and digestive organs). This is a very reasonable thing to do considering what Miss La Rue has told him. He knows from experience that looking in detail at her feet will not shed much light on sickness and other abdominal symptoms. However, he examines her mouth and hands as both these parts of the body can give clues to what's happening in the belly.

When he was at medical school he was taught to examine this part of the body in four stages.

1. Look.
2. Feel.
3. Percuss — that is to tap the abdomen in various places.
4. Listen — with a stethoscope.

He looks and sees a normal looking lady's abdomen. He makes a mental note that it might just be a little swollen below the belly button.

After warning Miss La Rue that his hands might be cold, and telling her to tell him if any place he feels hurts, he begins to gently feel the whole abdomen. He starts in the bottom left and goes anti-clockwise around. He will later make a note as following.

There seems to him to be a balloon shaped swelling below the belly button which arises out of the pelvis. This could be a full bladder.

'May I ask you when you last passed water Rita?'

'Just before I left home doctor — about fifteen minutes ago.'

The doctor then percusses (taps) the abdomen with his fingers. He finds a slightly dull mass where he felt the swelling.

He then listens with his stethoscope. The bowel is gurgling along quite happily. There is nothing else unusual. He then uses an electronic device to listen to the lower part of the abdomen. This is like a stethoscope with a microphone attached so much quieter sounds can be heard. He finds a regular tapping sound in the lower abdomen. He times this over thirty seconds and counts eighty 'taps'.

The doctor considers doing an internal examination. This involves him putting a disposable plastic glove on and gently inserting an examining finger into either the rectum or vagina. This kind of examination will often give a great deal of information about the lower pelvis. On this occasion the doctor feels he has all the information he needs, and so he thanks Miss La Rue, and goes back to his desk having asked her to get dressed.

At this stage of any examination the doctor will probably have a very good idea of what has brought the patient to the doctor. If he hasn't he may do further tests or write to a specialist for another opinion.

However, Dr Elton is fairly sure why Rita has felt sick and has a swollen abdomen. He remembers at medical school that he was taught that there were only five causes of an enlarged abdomen. They all began with the letter 'F'.

They were 1. Fat. 2. Flatus (air) 3. Fluid 4. Faeces (motion) and 5 which is what is affecting Miss La Rue.

He gently tells her what he suspects has happened. You may like to guess at the diagnosis yourself, and also decide what additional question needs to be asked and what test will confirm the diagnosis.

Miss La Rue is pregnant. The fifth 'F' stands for foetus (developing baby.) She tells the doctor that the first day of her last period was 1 January. As it is now nearly the middle of April, Rita is about fourteen weeks pregnant. A pregnancy test confirms the diagnosis. The 'tapping' sound heard with the electronic aid was the foetal heart. If the pregnancy goes ahead normally then the baby is due to be born on 9 October of that year. The total length of a human pregnancy is forty weeks.

In this case there is nothing 'wrong' with Rita. However, making the diagnosis is only the beginning of the help the doctor will be able to give her. He will discuss all the implications of being pregnant, and what having a baby could mean to her at this stage of her life.

He discussed the possibility of terminating the pregnancy with Rita. After everything has been explained to her she says she has thought about this, and she wishes to go ahead and have the baby.

> Termination of pregnancy, or abortion, is possible in certain circumstances. It is, however, not a procedure to enter into lightly. The law on abortion varies in different countries. In England, Wales, and Scotland two doctors must agree that there are sound reasons for this operation to be performed.

What a doctor writes in your medical notes is completely confidential and no-one sees them but the doctor. Doctors will never disclose anything from these notes without your consent. Our imaginary Doctor Elton has a computer for recording much of the routine medical matters – like lists of vaccinations – but this is what he wrote about Miss La Rue. As you can see much is in a form of shorthand which is usually yet another – if unintentional – protection of confidentiality.

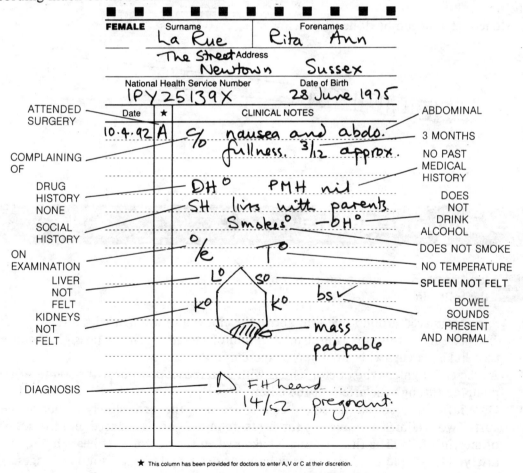

★ This column has been provided for doctors to enter A,V or C at their discretion.

FORM FP8

Tests

It may be that the doctor is not sure of the diagnosis after talking to you and making an examination. Often some tests are done.

Urine tests

Urine is a product filtered from the blood by the kidneys. As such it is often a very valuable guide to the internal workings of the body.

Modern testing can be done very easily and quickly using strips which are dipped into a sample of urine.

Blood tests

There are literally hundreds of tests that can be done on blood. The red cells can be measured. They may be small and pale in cases of anaemia when the body lacks iron. Too many white cells may indicate infection.

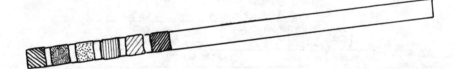

Blood pressure

Blood pressure is usually measured in the following way.

1. A cuff is placed around one arm above the elbow and inflated with air.
2. The pressure in this cuff is measured in mm of mercury. This is possible because a tube links the cuff with a column of mercury.
3. As the cuff tightens the doctor listens with a stethoscope to hear the sound of blood pumping through the artery at the elbow.
4. Once inflated − so that no sound can be heard − the air is slowly let out of the cuff. Two readings are taken as the pressure in the cuff is reduced and the column of mercury falls. The first reading is taken when the doctor first hears blood in the artery. The second is taken as the column of mercury falls and sound changes.

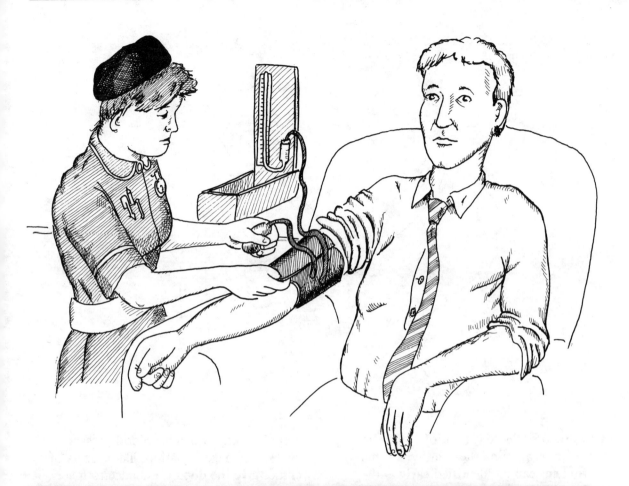

Stethoscope

The stethoscope is probably the instrument, along with a black bag, that most people associate with the doctor. It's basically a tube (or tubes) through which it is possible to listen to the internal workings of the body. With one you can hear the action of the heart, air going in and out of the lungs, and the bowels working.

The inventor of the stethoscope was a man called René Laennec. His first experiment was with a roll of paper. The first real stethoscopes were wooden cylinders. These days the tubes are made of rubber, and the sound is much clearer. You can easily make an old style stethoscope and hear the sounds that Laennec would have heard.

Place a cardboard tube – the centre of a toilet roll is ideal – on a friend's bare chest. The room should be quiet, as the sounds are not very loud. You'll hear the sounds 'lub-dub' repeated over and over again. These are the sounds of the heart's valves shutting.

Not only sick people are checked over

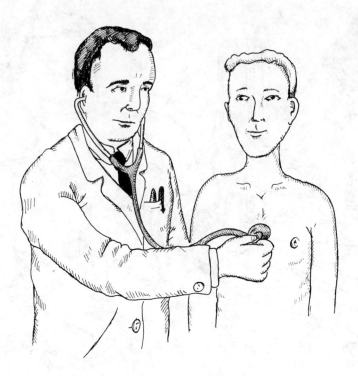

by doctors. There is a lot of emphasis now on examining the healthy, so that problems can be identified early and treated before they become serious. So children are checked before they go to school to see that they are developing normally. An adult's health check would include: weight; height; blood pressure check; urine examination. These sorts of clinics give the doctor a chance to meet the patient and give general advice like stopping smoking and cutting down an excessive alcohol intake.

How to get the most out of your doctor.

1. If you do not understand what the doctor has told you, or what he or she is doing to you, then ask.
2. Ask about any medicines you are given. It is quite reasonable to know how they will work, and what − if any − side effects there might be.
3. Non-urgent visits to the doctor are usually booked in advance. If you prefer one particular doctor in the practice, then ask for that person. If it is one of your parents who books the appointment then ask them to do this. Most practices have more than one doctor. If you would, for example, prefer to see a lady doctor then there shouldn't be any difficulty fixing this.

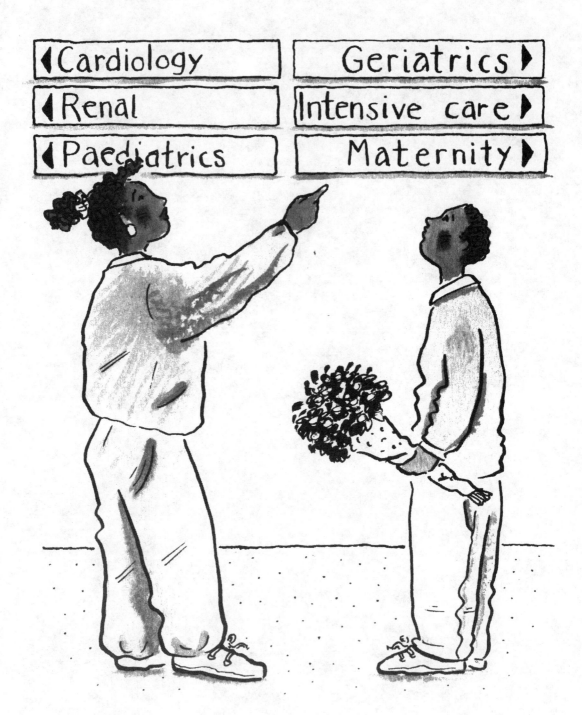

Hospital

Hospitals are places which care for the sick and wounded. However there are many different departments in a busy general hospital, and not all are concerned with illness. The maternity department, for example, looks after many fit healthy women who are having babies.

Hospitals are run by a team of people just as the family doctor's surgery is. In this hospital team there are: cleaners, clerks, consultants, cooks, dieticians, hospital administrators, junior doctors, laboratory technicians, laundry workers, midwives, nurses, pharmacists, porters, physiotherapists, radiographers, receptionists, social workers and telephonists.

Out-Patient Clinics

Most patients who go to hospital do not need to stay in overnight or longer. These clinics provide expert specialized opinions on patients whom the family doctor has sent up for a second opinion.

Within the hospital there are clinics which deal with many conditions.

Casualty

This is a department which deals with accidents and emergencies. Indeed it is often called the Department of Accident and Emergency Medicine. Many of the patients arrive by ambulance. The doctors and nurses have access to all the other facilities in the hospital.

Wards for Hospital In-Patients

There are beds on these units which care for patients who need to stay in hospital. This may be to look after them while they recover from an illness or operation, or so that tests can be carried out to determine why they are ill. Each ward is run by a sister (or charge nurse, if male). Each nurse will have work allocated to her (or him).

Laboratories

These are staffed by doctors and technicians who are able to undertake a whole variety of tests on such body fluids as blood and urine. They are able to look for germs that might be causing illness.

Many of the new developments in the science of medicine have been discovered and developed in hospital laboratories. Perhaps one of the most famous discoveries was that of penicillin in 1929. Sir Alexander Fleming found it almost by chance in the laboratory at St Mary's Hospital in London. He noticed that a bacteria he was growing in the laboratory had an area around it where the bacteria would not grow. A mould was growing in this area and when he experimented with this mould he found that it prevented the growth of bacteria, although it would not harm human cells. He called this mould penicillin.

A blood bank in the haematology laboratory stores blood until it is needed. (Blood kept like this has a shelf life of about three days.) Healthy donors have given the blood and the laboratory has run tests to determine the blood group. All the blood is stored until it is needed. Giving blood is painless. Eighteen is the minimum age that donors are accepted.

X-ray Department

Although there are many new ways of producing an image of the body, X-rays still remain one of the most important. X-rays can travel through the body, but are stopped by bone. Sometimes material is put into the body which will show up on an X-ray. A liquid made up with barium, for example, is opaque to X-rays and so outlines the stomach showing an ulcer which might be in its surface. Barium, which is harmless and not absorbed by the body, can also be given as an enema into the lower bowel, via the rectum, to produce an outline of the lower digestive tract.

Computerized Axial Tomography (CAT) scanners sometimes known as brain or body scanners take very special pictures using computers and these appear as if very detailed slices have been taken through the body. They present accurate images, not only of bones like X-rays, but also of softer tissue inside the body, for example the liver, which would not show up in detail on an X-ray.

Magnetic Resonance Imaging (MRI) uses magnetic fields and computers to build up cross-sectional images of the body. It is non-invasive and gives particularly good pictures of nervous tissue and joints.

Since X-rays were developed in 1895 these and many other ways have been devised to enable doctors to 'look' inside the human body and see what is going on.

A Dr Beaumont found one way of looking inside the body before the invention of X-rays. In 1822 a Canadian man called Alexis St Martin was shot in the side by a gun. He survived, but a 'window' was left into his stomach as the wound never closed. Dr Beaumont used this to peer into St Martin's stomach and to experiment with it. He lowered different foods into it on silk threads and timed how long each took to digest. He then took out the digestive juices and experimented with them. These experiments were often interrupted as St Martin kept running away, but they gave a great deal of important information to doctors of the time. Today flexible tubes can be passed into the mouth and down into the stomach to see what is happening and these days patients must give their consent to such experiments! The instruments used to do this are called endoscopes. They are about as thick as a finger and are made up of many fibre optic cables. These strands of glass will carry light and can bend, so that they give direct vision around 'corners' into many parts of the body which before had only been seen in life when surgeons made an incision to look in from the outside.

Not only can the doctor look with these instruments but they also can use them to take out (biopsy) parts of the body. Suppose a patient has a growth in his or her bowel. The surgeon can view it throught the endoscope then biopsy part of it. This can be sent to doctors in the pathology section of the laboratory, who specialize in the study of body disease (pathology). They will report exactly what the growth is. If it is a cancer it will be removed by the surgeon. If it is safe to leave (benign), then the endoscope has saved the patient an exploratory operation.

Sound waves are also used to produce images of the inside of a body. This is a safe way to check a baby is growing normally.

Lasers, narrow and very intense beams of light, are often used in hospitals. They can stop bleeding or even destroy a growth. Their accuracy makes them very useful in eye surgery. If a patient has a detached retina at the back of the eye, the eye surgeon can fire the laser at the tear and 'spot weld' it back into place.

Physiotherapy

This treatment improves mobility of patients. For instance, after some months in a leg plaster with a broken bone a patient can be taught exercises to strengthen leg muscles. Similarly a patient on a medical ward with a chest infection can be encouraged to cough up phlegm from the chest.

Speech Therapy

Speech therapists have a department in the hospital for treating speech problems such as stutters, and patients who have speaking difficulties after a stroke or throat operation.

Dieticians

Dieticians give advice about the most suitable foods to eat.

Pharmacy

All the drugs and medicines in the hospital come from the pharmacy. Each ward has a small trolley with patients' individual medicines. These are taken around by the nurses on their rounds.

Surgical Theatre

Surgeons perform operations within the hospital's operating theatre. Each day sees a schedule of operations which have been planned.

Newer ways of 'seeing' inside the body also play an important part in many operations today. Some heart surgery is a good example. Suppose a small artery supplying blood to the heart muscle itself becomes blocked. Today's heart specialist is able to pass a thin wire into it and guide it along inside the artery until it reaches the blockage. Then he or she can use the wire to break through the blockage and restore the flow of blood to the heart muscle. The whole operation can take place without the patient having to have any form of incision apart from a small cut in the groin to let the wire be fed into the artery.

Not all operations are planned, of course. Plenty are done as emergencies – like this one, which Sarah had when she was fifteen and developed an inflammation of the appendix. This is how she recorded what happened in her diary.

9.00 a.m.
Woke up with a belly ache that came and went. Felt sick. Edward [Sarah's younger brother)] ate my boiled egg. It's school holidays, so I stay in bed anyway.

Midday
Pain's getting worse. Felt sick. Was sick. Mum takes my temperature – 38°C – well up. She says she'll get the doctor later, if I'm not better.

3.00 p.m.
Pain's there all the time now. Been sick again. Pain's moved to right lower belly. Edward says it's wind. Just because he's always letting off.

5.30 p.m.
Dr Elton turns up. He's really old – about fifty – with cold hands. He asks lots of questions about the pain, takes my temperature and prods me about. Lots of 'ums' and 'ahs'. Doesn't say much, does Doc Elton. Then he tells Mum I've got appendicitis – needs an operation. Will it hurt? What happens if the anaesthetic doesn't work?

6.15 p.m.
Ambulance arrives and they cart me off on a sort of trolley. Mum's coming. She's got my overnight bag and some magazines. Edward starts to cry. He's only nine.

Ambulance shoots off without flashing lights. Every now and then the driver puts the siren on to get through the traffic. If the pain gets any worse my screams should do instead.

7.00 p.m.
Taken up to the ward. I'm stuck near the nurses' desk. A lot more docs in white coats. A lot younger than Doc Elton. And one only a bit older than me who's really wicked looking. I'll freak out if he comes to touch my belly.

8.00 p.m.
THREE doctors come and ask me all the same questions. When did the pain start? What's it like? (painful!) Does it come and go? When was my last period? And did I have

a boyfriend? (Mum said I hadn't.) Was I feeling sick and lots of questions about going to the loo.

Then they all felt me again. The dishy one did touch my belly! He turned out to be a medical student and the others all ignore him.

8.25 p.m.

An old doctor, called a registrar, came back with a nurse and stuck a finger up my bum. Asked if it hurt, and the nurse watched him do it! Said it helped him make up his mind if I needed an operation. It may have helped him, but it didn't do a lot for me.

9.05 p.m.

I'm for the operation. Had nothing to eat or drink for hours. There's a sign up above my head to say so. Like those signs you see above the cages at the zoo. I could be sick or something and choke on food during the anaesthetic a nurse said. Cheerful.

Mum signs the form to say it's OK to go ahead. I don't care − feel sleepy and happy after an injection to get me ready.

Can hardly keep awake as I'm wheeled off to the operating theatre. Felt a needle in the back of my hand. Someone said 'Just a small prick'. (Robert Jones told me a joke about this at school once.) Asleep before I could give them a witty reply.

6.00 a.m.

Woke up wondering where I am. A nurse is taking my blood pressure. (Learnt a LOT about hospitals yesterday.) As I'm writing this other nurse comes up and tells me all went well. She tells me the doctors took my appendix out just before it burst. Good old Dr Elton. My belly hurts a bit but nothing like yesterday. Don't feel like eating yet!

Later in the day Mum and Dad and Edward come and see me. Only two visitors at a time, but the ward sister says Edward doesn't count. (Knew that already.)

She says I'll be out of hospital in two or three days. The stiches will dissolve on their own, so no-one will have to take them out. In a year I'll hardly be able to see the scar!

Operations may also be done with the aid of a microscope. Developments in microsurgery have meant such operations as rejoining severed limbs are possible.

Using the microscope, delicate and minute nerves and blood vessels may be stitched back together.

Maternity Unit

A maternity unit is run by doctors and midwives who care for pregnant mothers. This unit is separate from the other wards and most of its patients are healthy. Babies who have been born prematurely (before the normal forty weeks of pregnancy) are looked after by paediatricians (specialists in children's medicine) within the protection of warm cots called incubators.

Intensive Care

The very sick may need intensive care for a while. This is given within a unit specializing in this treatment. There are many more staff for each patient than on the general wards. Machines may help the patient to breathe, and other instruments carefully and continually monitor the patient's condition.

With all these departments, an average district hospital will have about 600 beds for its patients. Some large hospitals are almost the size of a small town. They need a great deal of thought and money to make them run. Apart from all the medical services a busy hospital needs a small army of people to run its kitchens, laundry, the cleaning department, as well as a finance department to see everyone gets paid.

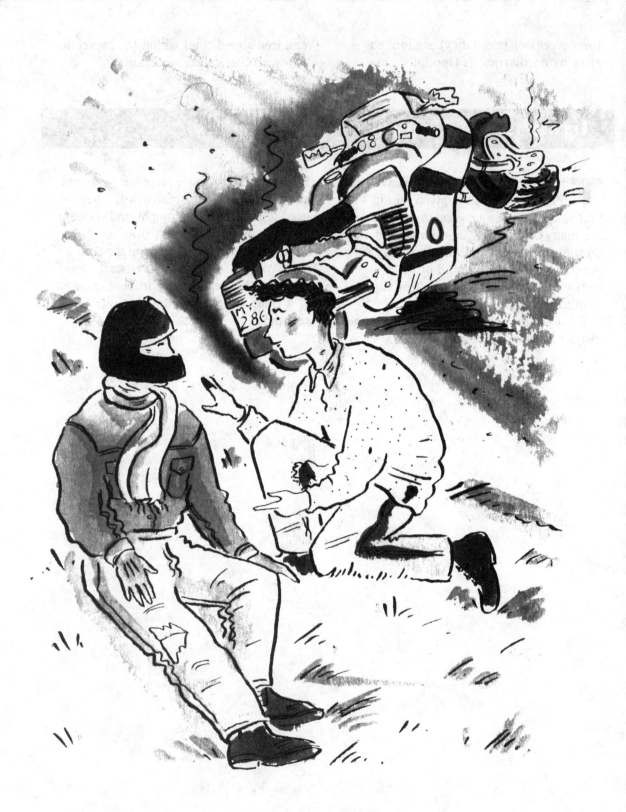

CHAPTER 7

First Aid

Practical lessons in first aid are the only real way to become a proficient first aider. Three voluntary organizations, the St John Ambulance, St Andrew's Ambulance Association, and the British Red Cross Society, all run first aid classes in Britain. You can find your local branch in the telephone book or the Yellow Pages.

First aid is the first help that is given to someone who has had an accident or who has suddenly become ill.

If you come across one of these situations there are three basic things to do:

1. Assess the situation and find out what has happened.
2. Give whatever assistance you can.
3. Get help.

1. It may be obvious what has happened. If a casualty has fallen off a motorbike and can't move his or her leg, he or she may be able to let you know which part of the body hurts. However, sometimes it is impossible to discover exactly what has happened at the scene.

Even so it is important to find out as much as possible from the victim or witnesses. This information should be passed on when expert help is available.

2. Once you have a diagnosis immediate treatment should be given. Remember your treatment should:

a. keep the casualty alive.
b. stop things getting worse.
c. help towards recovery.

Details of treatments are given in the following pages. Remember that a casualty may have more than one injury. In real life anything can happen in an accident or emergency.

It is important to take control of the situation in a kind but firm way. People who are sick or injured will be very frightened. So may friends or others who have witnessed a terrible event. Everyone feels better once any air of panic has been swept away.

3. Send for expert help and assistance. Do not delay any immediate life saving action to do this, but as soon as possible send someone to telephone 999 and alert the emergency services.

Remember not to come to any harm yourself. Look out in particular for such hazards as: fire, traffic, electric shock, thin ice and gas fumes.

3. The telephone is usually the best way to get emergency help.

● Dial or tap out 999. No money is needed.
● The person who answers will ask you which service you want. This is usually the ambulance, the fire brigade, or the police. In special circumstances you may need the coast guard or mountain rescue.
● Give your phone number.
● When through to the emergency service tell them:
    Who you are,
    What has happened.
    Where the problem is.
● Do not put the 'phone down until you are asked to.

There are three immediate threats to life:

1. When the air way is blocked off or the patient is not breathing.
2. When the heart has stopped.
3. When severe bleeding is happening.

(Severe bleeding (3) can be stopped by direct pressure. 1 and 2 are dealt with by emergency resuscitation.)

Resuscitation

If resuscitation is necessary it must be started as quickly as possible. The human brain can only survive without oxygen for around three minutes. It's easy to remember the three vital ingredients of this emergency treatment — easy as A B C:

A irway must be kept open to allow oxygen into the lungs.

B reathing must continue.

C irculation of the blood must occur so that oxygen is taken around the body. (And in particular to the brain).

Artifical respiration

This is sometimes quite rightly called the 'kiss of life'. It is performed on someone who has stopped breathing. Air is blown into their lungs.

First clear the airway if it is blocked. This may mean taking false teeth, vomit, chewing gum, a toy or any debris out of the mouth. Tilt the head backwards as shown so that the tongue is lifted forward and clear of the airway.

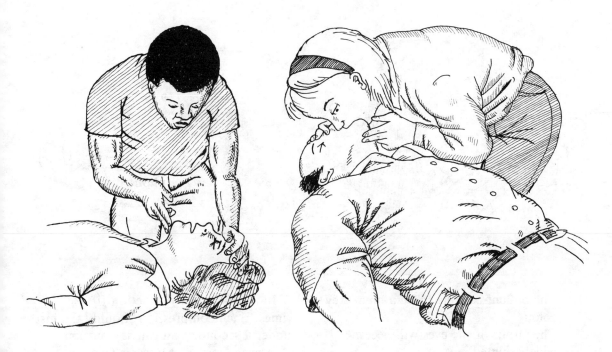

Second pinch the casualty's nostril shut and take a big breath in yourself. Blow this air into the patient's lungs as shown. The chest will rise as you do this. If it doesn't then adjust the position of the casualty's head to open the airway. (If it still does not rise then the airway may be blocked – treat as choking.)

After this first deep breath watch the casualty's chest fall as the air comes out. Then repeat the process a second time.

After these two breaths have been given check the casualty's pulse rate. If it is not felt go immediately to cardiac (heart) massage. (see page 76.)

If the heart is beating normally continue with the kiss of life with between sixteen to eighteen breaths per minute until normal breathing begins. When this happens place the casualty in the recovery position. (see page 77.)

Only do the kiss of life if a patient has stopped breathing. Do not try it on friends who are breathing normally.

Heart massage

If the heart is not beating then heart massage must be started. Check for heart-beat in the following way.

Feel for the carotid pulse in the neck. Turn the face to one side and feel the groove alongside the adam's apple. If the heart has stopped beating no pulse will be felt. Also:

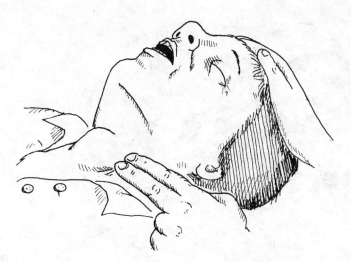

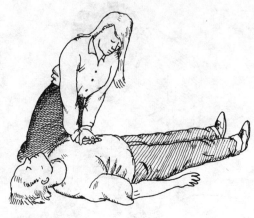

1. The patient is likely to be a blue/grey colour.
2. The pupils of the eyes will become widely dilated.

THIS TECHNIQUE IS DANGEROUS IF THE HEART HAS NOT STOPPED. MAKE SURE THAT YOU KNOW HOW TO TELL IT HAS.

With cardiac massage you will be doing the pumping work of the inactive heart. Therefore it is important to position your two hands directly over the heart.

1. The patient is flat on his or her back and you are to one side.
2. Place the heel of one hand on the lower half of the breast bone.
3. Place the heel of the other hand on top.
4. Straighten your arms and rock your body forwards pressing the adult patient's breast bone about four centimetres down.

This action will compress the heart and expel blood from it. So circulation is restarted artifically.

In adults repeat this action fifteen times. Each compression should take just under a second. You can say out loud 'Massage One ... Massage Two ... Massage Three ...' Saying those words will take just under three seconds.

After fifteen compressions – if you are on your own – move to the head and perform two 'breaths' as above in the 'kiss of life'. Keep this cycle of two breaths and fifteen compressions going and check for a pulse in the neck about every three minutes. Keep this up until the heart beat begins again and breathing starts. Then place the casualty in the recovery position.

With children it is necessary to use less pressure but do more compressions. You can learn these at First Aid classes.

If there are two of you, one performs the heart massage and the other performs the lung inflations.

The first aider should watch for signs that the procedure is succeeding – that is that the pulse returns and the patient's colour improves as blood with oxygen begins to circulate.

Recovery Position

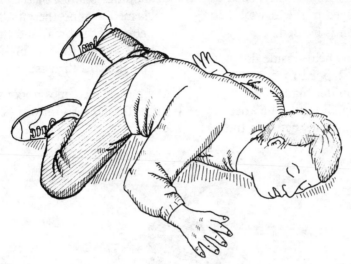

This position is for the care of an unconscious person. In it the tongue falls forward and not back where it might block the airway to the lungs. Similarly any vomit from the stomach will run out of the mouth rather than back into the lungs. There is a real danger of both of these happening if an unconscious person is left on his or her back.

You need to practise turning the body onto its side like this. The head should be to one side not face down.

DO NOT MOVE ANYONE WHO MAY HAVE A SPINAL INJURY. Movement may damage the delicate spinal cord within the bones of the spine.

You may suspect a broken spine if the casualty complains of neck or back pains after a serious accident. If the spinal cord is damaged the patient may feel 'dead' below the level of that damage. For example, a break in the spine of the lower back will result in feeling and movement being absent in the legs. An injury higher up in the neck may result in similar loss of movement and sensation in the arms.

Choking

This emergency is so well known it hardly needs description. As well as the 'choking' sign, the patient will be unable to talk, and usually grasps his or her throat.

- The patient's own cough will often clear the airway.
- If you suspect a foreign body, such as a sweet, has lodged in the airway then immediate action is needed:

1. Infants should be held upside down by the legs and slapped firmly between the shoulder blades

2. Children may be laid over the knee and slapped four times between the shoulder blades.

3. Adults should be slapped between the shoulder blades, or they can be clasped around the middle, from behind (as shown) and the fist can be used to give four quick hard inward and upward thrusts.

If the patient becomes unconscious then begin artificial respiration. (The 'kiss of life'.)

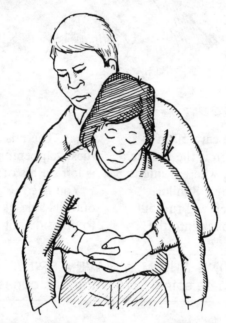

Broken bones [Fractures]

Fractures may be open (when the skin is broken) or closed (when it is not). This is an important distinction since germs can enter an open fracture and lead to additional serious complications. It is not always easy to decide if a bone is broken — even with X-rays. However, here are some guide lines for the first aider. Some of these may seem obvious but they are surprisingly easy to forget in an emergency:

- Broken bones are usually painful, especially on movement. (Beware of fractured hips in the elderly as these may be painless.)

- The patient tends not to use the affected area. Not many people walk when they have a broken leg.
- The area looks deformed or may move in an unusual way – like a bird with a broken wing.
- Broken bones often have a large amount of swelling around the fracture. So treat injuries as fractures if there is any doubt.
- The ends of broken bones can sometimes be heard grating together like the edges of a broken biscuit.

Treatment

General rule – the more immobile the fracture is, the less likely is further damage. For example, converting a closed fracture to an open one. So you must use your common sense to prevent the fractured bones from moving – perhaps by using some kind of splint or bandage. You can learn these techniques at First Aid classes.

Wasps and Bee Stings

If the sting is still in the person's skin then it should be removed. It can be picked out with tweezers, grasping the sting as close to the skin as possible. Or 'brushed off' using the back of a kitchen knife. It is important not to squeeze the poison sac further.

Then wash the area with cold water.

A wet compress should relieve the itching. Calamine lotion is also effective against the irritation.

Burns and Scalds

Burns may be caused by hot objects (dry burns), hot liquids and steam (scalds), by chemicals, electricity, and friction. (e.g. rope burns from sliding down a rope).

The two most important things to look for when assessing how severe a burn is are:

1. How much of the surface of the body is affected: head = 9%, arm = 9%, leg = 18%, front of torso = 18%, back of torso = 18%. These figures of either 9 or 18 are easy to remember. The palm of your hand is about 1%. The more surface area burnt, the more serious is the injury.

2. How deep the burns are.

   All electrical burns and all burns bigger than the size of a postage stamp – should be seen by a doctor. Deep burns are not particularly painful because the nerve endings will have been destroyed.

Minor superficial burns can be treated by running the burn under cold water. After this cover the burn with a clean dry dressing. Do not prick any blisters that form as this could allow germs into the wound and cause infection.

Fainting

A faint is a loss of consciousness caused by lack of blood and oxygen to the brain. Fainting is the body's way of improving that blood supply. You faint and fall down and the blood runs to the head. There are lots of causes such as: a fright, sudden pain, tiredness or standing still for a long time in hot weather.

If a person begins to feel faint, lay them down on the floor, and lift their legs up. If they do faint, lay them in the recovery position, and make sure there is nothing tight around the neck.

As they recover, reassure them and sit them up gradually. Check for any signs of injury from falling.

Epileptic Fit

These are quite common and can look most alarming. There are usually four stages to a major epileptic fit:

1. The patient falls to the ground often giving a short cry.
2. The patient then becomes rigid and the face becomes dark blue/red for a few seconds.
3. There is then a stage of convulsions, in which the body's muscles contract.
4. There is then a state of quiet relaxation and the patient may look asleep.

The aim for the first aider is to prevent the patient hurting him-or herself. So try and catch the body before the fall if possible. When the person is on the floor clear away anything, such as furniture, which it would be possible to bang into during the convulsion.

Loosen any tight clothing around the neck.

In the fourth, 'quiet' stage of the fit lay the patient in the recovery position.

Report the fit to a doctor unless the person is a known epileptic and has had similar uncomplicated fits before. People who have epilepsy often carry a warning bracelet or card.

Sometimes a young child who develops a high temperature may fit. Report these types of fits to a parent and get medical help immediately.

Bleeding and Wounds

Wounds to the body vary a great deal. Some common types which the first aider will encounter are:

1. Clean cuts of the skin.
2. Torn lacerated skin from such things as barbed wire and dog bites. These wounds are often dirty.
3. Bruises. These are caused by blows to the body, after which bleeding occurs underneath the skin to give the characteristic bruise.
4. Stab wounds. Injuries such as a garden fork in the foot have a small entry hole but may have caused a deep and dirty wound with much internal damage.

All these wounds cause bleeding. Along with either the heart or breathing stopping, a big haemorrhage (bleed) is a life threatening event. Of course not all bleeds endanger life.

> Direct pressure is always the first step to control any bleeding.

1. The first thing to do with a bleeding wound is to stop the flow of blood. This is done by direct pressure. So press the cut with a clean handkerchief or towel. After five minutes most minor wounds will have stopped bleeding.
2. Wash the wound with clean water. It is important to remove any dirt from the wound.

Larger cuts may need stitches in them. Other wounds such as stab wounds or lacerations are treated in a similar way. Remember they are more likely to contain dirt than a 'clean' cut. Also, it is important to be aware that a heavy blow causing a bruise, or a stab wound with a small entry site may cause more serious problems such as internal bleeding which may not be visible.

A scalp wound may bleed alarmingly. Do not poke or probe a scalp wound. Apply a dressing larger than the wound and bandage it on firmly.

Shock

Heavy bleeding is one cause of shock. In the state of shock vital areas of the body fail to receive blood. Signs of shock to look for are:

1. Pale skin which is cold and clammy.
2. Patient may complain of feeling faint and sick.
3. Pulse rate is fast and weak.
4. Breathing is fast and shallow.

Shock may be caused by severe pain or

the mental shock of something very unpleasant happening.

Shock may be the result of loss of body fluids, such as blood loss, fluid loss from severe diarrhoea, or plasma loss from burns to the skin.

The second cause of shock is the most serious form.

What to do with a patient in shock

1. Lay the patient down and give reassurance.

2. Keep the patient warm and comfortable while arranging for urgent help to come.
3. If possible deal with the cause of shock, e.g. stop any bleeding.
4. Do not move patient unless necessary. If vomiting or unconsciousness seems likely, place in recovery position.
5. Do not give anything to eat or drink.

Nose Bleeds

Nose bleeds are usually stopped by doing the following:

1. Sit the person down with the head forward and the mouth open. Ask the patient to spit any blood out, and breathe through the mouth.
2. Pinch the soft part of the nose for ten minutes.
3. After ten minutes the bleeding should have stopped. If it hasn't then repeat the process.
4. Advise the person not to blow the nose for several hours. This could disturb the clot that has formed and restart the bleed.

Nose bleeds that continue despite these efforts should be seen by a doctor.

Drowning

The treatment for drowning is to get air into the lungs and to restart breathing if it has stopped. (See resuscitation and 'kiss of life' mentioned earlier.)

Patients should be taken to hospital as quickly as possible as water in the lungs can produce various complications.

Always continue artifical resuscitation of 'drowned' patients as recovery is still possible after long periods of immersion and after apparent 'death'.

Poisoning

People may be poisoned either deliberately or by accident. Poisons have usually been taken by mouth. However, poisons may be inhaled, injected, or, as in the cases of some farm pesticides, absorbed through the skin.

Follow these steps to give first aid to someone who has been poisoned.

1. If the person is unconscious place in the recovery position. Be prepared to begin resuscitation. If the person is conscious ask what poison has been taken.
2. Keep the casualty comfortable, warm and dry, and give reassurance.
3. Get medical help urgently, while watching that the patient's condition does not deteriorate. Many poisons, including alcohol, may depress breathing.

DO NOT make the patient sick in an effort to bring the poison out of the stomach. If this has to be done it needs an expert to do it. Some poisons, for example petroleum products, can cause further harm if the patient is sick.

The hospital will need the following information from you:

1. Name and age of the person.
2. What drug or poison you think may have been taken.
3. What time that poison was taken.
4. Any empty medicine bottles, or vomit, or if, for example, a young child has taken 'red berries', then a sample of that bush, tree or plant.
5. A note of any events such as the patient being sick.

All medicines and dangerous substances such as weed killers or bleaches should be kept safe in a safe place where young children cannot get hold of them.

Electric shock

Electric shocks can come from many sources, including railway lines, lightning and the power supply in the home.

The first consideration when dealing with someone who has had an electric shock is *not* to have two victims. So the source of electricity must be switched off if there is any danger that the person is still 'live'. If necessary this may mean waiting for someone from the electricity board. In the home it is fairly easy to turn off a switch, or pull out a plug or, if you know how to, turn off the electric supply to the whole house.

WHEN it is safe:

1. Check the patient is breathing. The usual procedures for resuscitation then apply. If unconscious leave in the recovery position.

2. Keep the patient warm.
3. Do not leave the patient but arrange for someone to get help fast.

Hypothermia

This is a dangerous lowering of the body temperature. In young people the usual cause is exposure to cold, wet and wind on a camping trip or hiking expedition. The elderly are at risk from it in the winter in their own home, as their bodies react to cold less well than the young. Very young babies also need special protection from the cold.

The signs of hypothermia are a drowsy, weak, cold patient who is often confused and speaking with a slurred voice. In severe cases the person may be unconscious and appear to be in a deep sleep or even dead.

Treatment aims to warm the patient up *slowly*. So cover him or her with something like a blanket or sleeping bag. If out in the open, it is particularly important to protect the casualty from the chilling effect of the wind.

> Do not use hot water bottles or electric blankets. A sudden rise in temperature can kill the hypothermic patient.

If conscious give sips of warm drinks, but *not* alcohol, because alcohol causes blood to move to the skin. This will cause more heat loss.

Head injury

A blow to the bony skull can cause injuries in various ways. The skull may break. A heavy blow may shake the brain up so much that consciousness is lost. Such an injury to the brain is called concussion.

Someone who has been knocked out should be placed in the recovery position. They should see a doctor as soon as possible to check that no serious brain damage has occurred.

A particularly tricky part of the skull to injure is the area above each ear. Blows here may be very serious which is why cricketers often wear helmets to protect themselves.

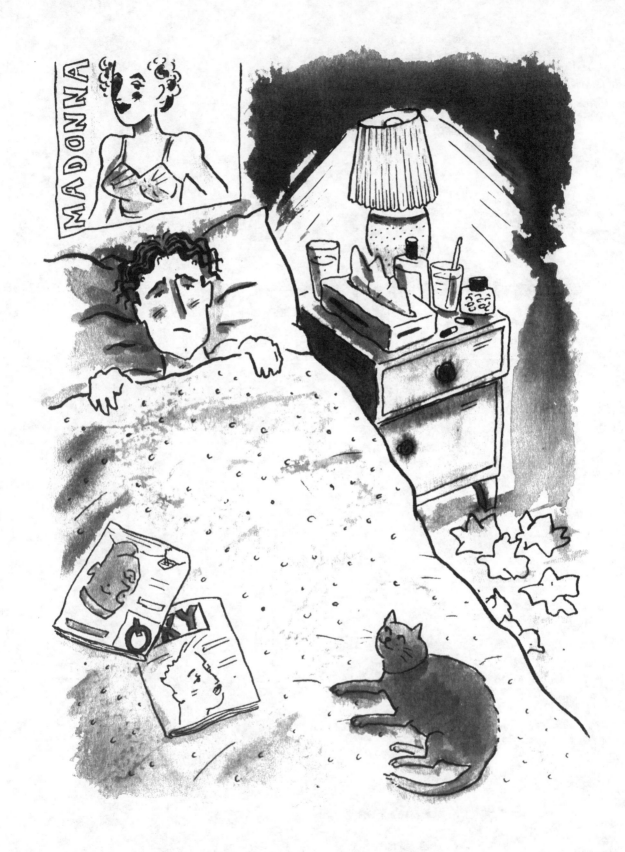

CHAPTER 8

Treatments

The dictionary defines 'treatment' as a way of dealing with, or behaving towards a person or thing. This is a pretty wide definition. As far as health and medical matters go most people's idea of treatment is a couple of paracetamol tablets and staying in a warm bed.

However, 'treatment' can vary from a medicine taken by mouth or plastering a broken bone, to recommending certain foods or wearing glasses. And an important thing about treating a medical problem is that very often doing nothing is the best treatment of all. One doctor advised me when I first qualified that the art of medicine was keep patients happy until nature made them better.

Medicines

There are thousands of different medicines. They may ease pain, make breathing easier, or cure an infection. There isn't, of course a pill for every ill. However, modern medicine has got some pretty amazing drugs to help sick people get better.

Medicines and their uses are always changing. As recently as the last century tomato ketchup was considered an excellent medicine for a whole host of diseases! Who knows what your children will be putting on their hamburgers.

There are several methods of administering medicines:

Creams and ointments. These medicines are rubbed into the skin.

Tablets and capsules. This is a common way of taking a medicine by mouth.

Inhalers. Drugs – such as those for asthma and the lungs – can be very quickly and effectively delivered by inhalation.

Injections. Medicine which cannot be taken by mouth may have to be injected.

Eye drops.

Suppository. This form of taking medicine is often joked about. However, putting a soft bullet shaped suppository inside the rectum can be very effective. If someone is being sick the suppository is inserted and melts with the heat of the body. The actual drug is then absorbed.

It is important to follow the instructions given with a medicine. Let's assume you have been given an antibiotic by your doctor for a sore throat. Take a look at the label. It should have your name, the date, how to take the medicine and the name of the antibiotic.

SHAKE THE BOTTLE
18/11/92
THE MIXTURE

One 5 ml. spoonful to be taken 3 times a day

Penicillin V
elixir BP
Please complete
course
Julia Gaylor

**Dr. P. A. LEFTLEY &
Dr. P. A. ROWAN**
Pulham Market, DISS, Norfolk
Tel. Pulham Market 227

Here are some ways familiar drugs work and what they are doing:

Reduce symptoms but not 'cure' – aspirin, paracetamol, antacids.

Replace something that's missing – insulin, iron.

Cure – antibiotics.

Deliberately given as a preparation for something else – anaesthetics.

Taken for their pleasurable effect – caffeine.

Taken to block a normal process or reaction in the body which is unwanted – antihistamine, contraceptive pill.

Taken to prevent illness – asthma inhaler, anti-malarials.

Aspirin and paracetamol

These are widely used pain killers, which dull pain and reduce inflammation. In addition they may lower raised body temperature.

Antibiotics

There are a great number of antibiotics. Penicillin is probably the best known. There are two basic ways that they work. Some antibiotics, like penicillin, kill bacteria. Others, like tetracycline, stop the bacteria growing.

Anaesthetics

These work in two ways. Local anaesthetics block nerves and prevent pain sensation passing to the brain of the fully conscious patient. General anaesthetics work in very complex ways and produce a complete, yet safe and controllable loss of consciousness in a patient.

Many general anaesthetics act in a similar way to alcohol. In fact, alcohol was used for centuries to give some form of anaesthetic during painful operations. It has many drawbacks though; it is difficult to get the dose exactly correct, it makes patients sick, and predicting how long the patient will be 'out' is nearly impossible.

In contrast, modern general anaesthetics work quickly, have predictable effects, and are easily reversed when the operation is complete. However, when alcohol was the only drug available it was better to be 'dead drunk' while your leg was being amputated on a medieval battle field than to be wide awake.

Antacids

Given that the hydrochloric acid in your stomach could burn a hole in some carpets, it is not surprising that many people get indigestion from time to time. Antacids work by attempting to neutralize some of this acidity.

Insulin

This is a hormone produced naturally by the body in the pancreas gland. It controls sugar levels in the blood. Without it, sugars such as glucose are neither used to give energy, nor stored in body cells for later use. When this happens the sugar spills over into the urine from the blood. This condition, where lack of natural insulin allows sugar to be lost in the urine, is called sugar

diabetes or diabetes mellitus. The missing insulin can be replaced by daily injections. (It can't be given by mouth because the stomach acid would destroy it.)

Not all diabetics need insulin. Some, mainly older people, can get by on tablets or just by being careful about what they eat.

Antihistamines

Histamine is a body chemical which is involved in the process of inflammation. When a nettle stings the skin and produces the familiar nettle rash, histamine is the chemical behind that reaction. It is also behind many allergies. Antihistamine drugs suppress that reaction, so they can be very helpful to those with hay fever. They suppress the action of histamine in the nose, for example, and they may stop it running.

Iron

Most people get enough iron for their body's needs from diet. Sometimes this supply needs boosting and then iron can be taken by mouth. It is not given in its basic form, as iron filings would not be absorbed. A common medicinal form is iron (ferrous) sulphate.

WARNING. All medicines are potential poisons if taken in the wrong dose or by the wrong people.

1. Follow the instructions.
2. Never take anyone else's medicines.
3. Finish the complete course.

Surgery

Surgery literally means the treatment of disease with the hands. It wasn't until the mid-nineteenth century when anaesthetics and ways of preventing infection were both discovered that surgery took off as a medical speciality. Before then surgery was too painful and too risky to be a popular form of treatment.

Surgery can be performed as an emergency. An example of this is the removal of an inflamed appendix as described on page 69. However, much surgery is carefully planned. The surgeon arrives for work in the morning and a list of operations for that day has been arranged. These patients then take their turn to be operated on in the operating theatre.

Within the speciality of surgery there is even more specialization. Orthopaedic surgery is concerned with bones and joints and includes dealing with fractures and dislocations.

Plastic surgery deals with the repair of damaged tissue. Some of it is cosmetic, but it isn't simply confined to vanity, such as giving a film star a more appealing shaped nose. Plastic surgeons are involved with treatment after burns, where skin is grafted to the wound. This not only keeps scarring to a minimum, it also protects the burn against infection.

Dental surgery involves looking after teeth and the mouth. Orthodontics deals with misplaced or crooked teeth. These are often moved back into the correct position with a metal brace fitted to the teeth.

Other surgery involves the surgeon working on the brain, or the chest or the kidneys.

Alternative Medicine

There are many other sorts of treatments. Some of these are what are called 'alternative' medicine. They are not usually given by the family doctor, but can go hand-in-hand and complement conventional treatments.

Acupuncture

Acupuncture involves a skilled person sticking fine metal needles into the body at various points. These may then be rotated or charged with a small electrical current. Some practitioners do not find it necessary to move the needles at all.

Acupuncture has been known in the Orient for thousands of years. Practitioners then spoke of a life force in the body which flowed along invisible lines called meridians. They believed that needles inserted along these lines could effect the balance between the two life forces known as 'Yin' and 'Yang'. Those with the skill would know exactly where to insert the needle. It may well be a distance from the actual problem. So, someone with a liver illness might have the needle inserted in their foot. Or a needle in the hand could be used to treat a headache.

There is no doubt that acupuncture works for some people. Western doctors began to take notice of the technique when they saw patients in China having operations, such as appendicectomy, after receiving acupuncture and without conventional anaesthetics.

Some Western doctors believe that the needles work, for example against pain, by stimulating the body to produce its own natural painkillers called endorphins. Most respected practitioners of acupuncture simply admit that they do not know how it works. It just does.

There is much to learn yet about this technique. Do not try it yourself. Acupuncture takes a lot of training and can be very dangerous in unskilled hands.

Homeopathy

Homeopathy is based on the idea that like cures like. It was founded in Europe about 200 years ago. A homeopathic doctor sees his work as an extension of conventional medicine. He or she will place great emphasis on treating the 'whole' patient. So, for example, the patient's personality is important in deciding treatment.

The basic idea behind homeopathic treatment is that if a drug in large doses produces symptoms similar to those produced by an illness, then very small doses of that drug will actually be effective in treating that illness. The aim of the homeopathic doctor is to get patients better rather than just relieve symptoms.

One example of 'like for like' would be splashing cold water on the face after waking up on a cold morning. Most would agree this is invigorating. However, a more obvious 'treatment' would be to splash *hot* water on the face on a cold morning. This might seem to be logical, but any benefit would obviously only be temporary.

Osteopathy

Osteopathy is based on manipulation of the muscles and joints of the body. Special attention is directed to the spine. Modern osteopaths believe that many symptoms, such as back ache, are caused when bones, muscles and joints are not working together in harmony. So, once the root of the problem has been identified by a skilled examination, manipulation of that part of the body can produce a return to normal function and give relief of the symptoms.

Some osteopaths go further and claim to be able to relieve symptoms such as headache and stomach pains by manipulation of joints.

Hypnotherapy

Hypnotherapy is a form of suggestion. The hypnotherapist uses, amongst other things, the sound of his or her voice to put the patient into a relaxed state of mind. In this 'trance' the patient will often disclose the root cause of a problem which, without hypnosis, he or she would not be able to reveal.

Hypnosis may be very effective in treating certain problems. These are often related to stress or anxiety. However, physical problems such as warts have been shown to go away after this has been suggested to the patient.

No-one knows for certain how hypnosis works. Some people cannot be be hypnotized. Some people are much more susceptible than others.

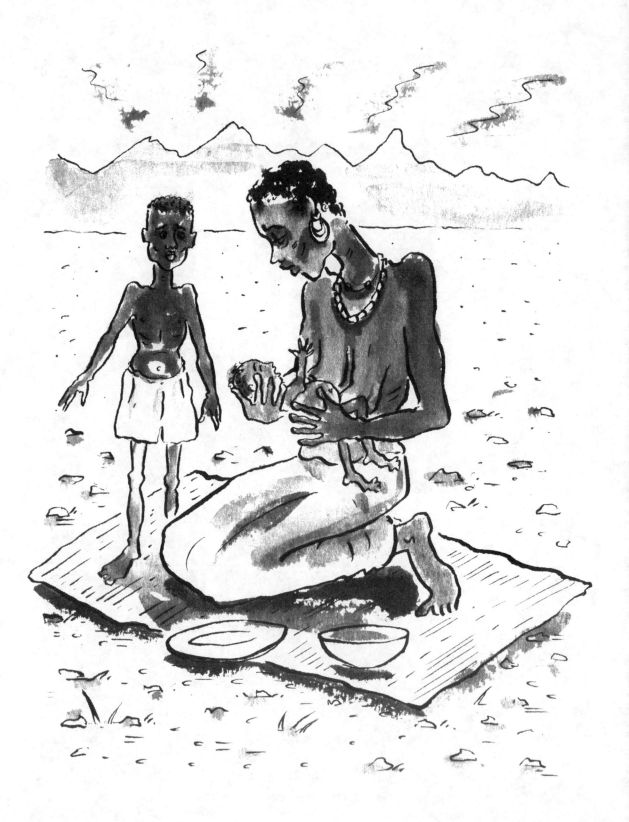

World Health and the Environment

Each year in England and Wales over 250,000 people die of diseases related to hardening of the arteries. These diseases include conditions such as heart attacks and strokes. In the United Kingdom these disorders of the circulation are by far the commonest causes of death.

It is easy to forget that the situation in many other parts of the world is very different to this. As we battle to keep our weight down, eat a healthy diet and stop smoking and drinking excessively, people elsewhere are dying in millions at an early age from very different problems.

It has been reliably estimated that in the UK 180,000 people die from disease which could have been prevented by healthy eating.

Just as many of the problems of western health are preventable, so are diseases in the Third World.

Malaria is one of the most important diseases of mankind. The problem is a very good example of how Third World health problems may be tackled, and also of the special problems posed for organizations like the World Health Organization who lead the fight against disease, poverty, and lack of health information.

The parasite that causes malaria is spread by mosquitoes. There are 200,000,000 cases of malaria a year, and of these 1,000,000 people will die. This makes malaria one of the commonest causes of death and sickness in the world.

Once the parasite is in the human body it is carried in the blood to organs such as the liver where it multiplies. After two weeks, or even longer, it returns to the blood stream and invades the circulating red cells. This causes the red cells to burst, and the parasites then move on to destroy others. It is at this stage that the victim first experiences the symptoms of headache and high fever.

As red cells are destroyed the infected person becomes more and more anaemic. Patients may recover after several bouts of fever, but children especially may become weaker and weaker. They may then die from a trivial illness which would not have caused serious problems if they had been in good health.

These are the ways malaria can be tackled:

1. Treat every person who has malaria. Although the mosquito will still bite humans it would not spread the parasite because no-one would have it in their blood to be spread.

     This is the situation in Europe where the malaria mosquito (Anopheles) does still exist.
2. The malaria mosquito can be prevented from biting. It can be killed with sprays, and nets can be fitted over beds. It is possible to avoid the bite simply by wearing long sleeved shirts and avoiding the time (early evening) and the places (damp and wet) when and where the mosquito is active.
3. People who are at risk from malaria may take drugs which prevent the disease getting a hold on their body even if they are bitten.

If you go on holiday to parts of the world where malaria exists, then you may have to take small doses of this preventative medicine while you are away. It is very important to take it as prescribed. For example, it needs to be continued for a while *after* returning. This is because the malaria parasite can emerge from organs such as the liver and this may occur in the weeks after you are back in Europe. Malaria is a good example of how the world can, and does try to tackle ill health, and the problems this poses. Here is a condition which can be both prevented and treated, yet kills a million people every year.

In Africa, for example, malaria has been wiped out of large towns. These are now safe. However, much money, time and staff would be needed to regularly treat the mosquito's breeding places in the country, and these resources are simply not available.

The good news is that the day may not be far away when we have a vaccine against malaria.

Three procedures would transform health in underdeveloped countries. They are things we often take for granted:

● Good sanitation.
● An effective immunization programme.
● Good nutrition.

Sanitation

We often take for granted being able to have an efficient toilet and being able to wash whenever we wish to. However, there is a very sophisticated system to deal with the bath water when the plug is pulled, and with the contents of the toilet when it is flushed.

Many countries do not have the money and resources to have efficient plumbing and sanitation systems. The waste may go straight into a river from which people draw drinking water. This can cause many different illnesses. Cholera, which leads to life threatening diarrhoea is one, and polio, which can cause muscular paralysis and death, is another. It is possible to be vaccinated against many of these illnesses. However for the reasons that these countries do not have efficient sewage disposal systems, they also do not have efficient immunization programmes.

Immunization

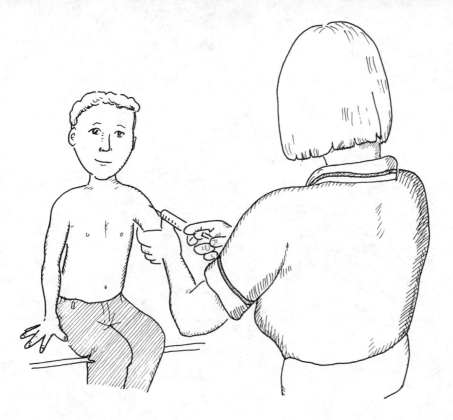

Immunization is one of the most important ways in which illness can be prevented. The doctor gives the patient a vaccine. This usually means giving a modified and harmless version of a germ which stimulates the patient's body to produce defences against that germ. These defences will be ready if the real germ comes along.

Nutrition

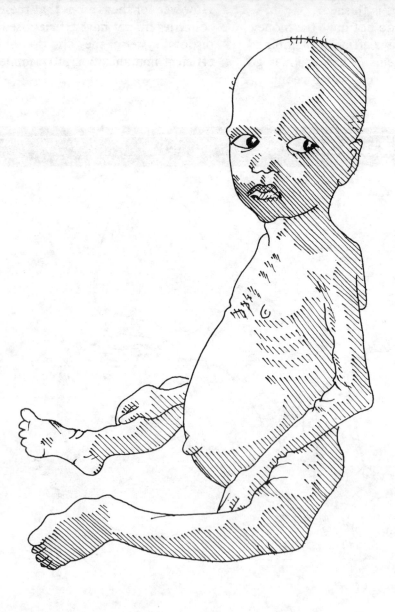

A good diet is necessary for good health. Poor nutrition results in poor health. Many thousands of children in the world are dying while you read this because they do not have enough food to eat.

The African child pictured here is ill because of poor diet. The condition is known as 'kwashiorkor' and is a word widely used in medicine to describe young children with a special kind of malnutrition. The child is wizened and shrunken. The muscles are weak and poorly developed. The belly often sticks out as gas swells up in the bowel underneath the weak abdominal muscles.

The term 'kwashiorkor' is a word used by the Ga tribe who live in Ghana. It means 'sickness the older child gets when the next baby is born'. This happens when, after a long period of breast feeding, a child is put onto the traditional family diet because a new born baby needs to be breast fed. The family diet is poor and the child develops 'kwashiorkor'. The child's new diet is low in protein because of a lack of good farming techniques, poor land to grow food crops, and general poverty. Malnutrition is the result.

This is not to say that basic diets are bad for you. In the western world many people have become ill through eating a poor diet. People who eat a basic well balanced diet are likely to avoid a whole range of conditions which affect the 'developed' countries. Heart attacks, for example, that result from eating high fat foods, are rare in Third World communities.

Television pictures have brought home to many people how different the lives of millions of people are in the Third World. However, you really have to visit these people to experience just how desperate things can be.

Recently I was travelling in one of the poorest countries of the world. In the countryside away from the towns, the adults can only expect to live to just over forty years of age. Also I saw many young babies who did not have names. I asked the mothers about this, and they told me that so many children died during the first year of life, that they preferred to wait until their first birthday before they named the infants.

The number of children who die within the first year of life is an indicator of the general standards of health within a community. Health workers usually express this figure as number of deaths per thousand. In a country with good health facilities this figure should be well under ten deaths per thousand.

In many poor countries this figure runs into hundreds for every thousand babies born.

Environment

The environment effects peoples' health all around the world. Whether pollution comes from cigarette smoke, the exhaust of a car, or an oil spill at sea, the end result to health is the same.

Mercury poisoning is an example of how the human body can be poisoned. Here are three 'case histories'.

'Mad as a hatter'. At one time workers in the hat industry used dyes to colour the hats. These dyes had mercury in them. This slowly accumulated in the 'hatters' bodies until they began to shake uncontrollably and in severe cases went mad. (Lewis Carroll may have used this idea for his Mad Hatter in *Alice in Wonderland*.)

In quite recent times fishing families around Minimata Bay in Japan began to suffer very severely with an illness which was eventually diagnosed as mercury poisoning. The source was eventually traced back to a factory which had discharged mercury waste into the bay. This mercury had passed up the food chain from small plant-eating fish to large fish such as tuna. These had then been caught and eaten by the unsuspecting fishermen.

Many cases of mercury poisoning have occurred in Pakistan and Guatemala when poor families have eaten grain treated with mercury. The mercury is used to treat the seed against fungal attack before it is sown. However, the peasants could not read these warnings and ate the seed.

The dangers of inhaling asbestos dust were described in the 1900s. In the 1930s it was realized what a danger asbestos was in the work place. Health suffered not only in asbestos mines, but also where the asbestos was used − for example in ship yards as fireproofing and insulation.

In the first century AD the Roman historian and scientist Pliny wrote that the weavers of the wicks for the lamps of the vestal virgins wore masks to protect their lungs. (Asbestos was used in making these wicks.) So, before he died in the eruption of Vesuvius, Pliny was giving an early warning about asbestos in the work place.

There are many other places of work such as mines, chemical plants, and nuclear power stations where, unless great care is taken, the environment can severely damage health − even in a hospital.

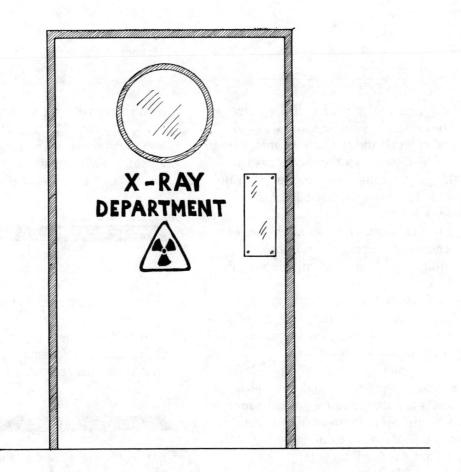

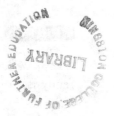

Now that you've read what Dr Peter Rowan has to say about the way our bodies work and the various things that can be done to get them better when things go wrong, why not read his fun guide to keeping your body healthy – *Body Wise*?

In this he turns the spotlight on the benefits of keeping fit and healthy by eating a good diet and enjoying regular exercise.

But *Body Wise* isn't just for food freaks and fitness fanatics. It's a book for everyone, whatever your shape and whatever shape you're in.

In it you can follow the *Body Wise* exercise programme, find out which sports and exercises are going to suit you best and discover why eating a healthy diet doesn't mean eating a boring diet.

Topics covered include:

Fit For Life

If you've ever wondered what fitness really is, you'll find the answer here.

You'll also find out why exercise will make you look better, feel better and give you a chance of living longer. And there's a health questionnaire to find out how health conscious you really are.

Your Body Type

We all have different bodies and different minds, and it would be a dull world if everyone was the same. Knowing the type of sports and exercises best suited to your own body type is a key step to enjoying them. Use Dr Rowan's Body Test to help find your own answer.

Food For Sport

Eating the right food is a major part of enjoying sport and doing well at what you do. Understanding what food contains and why our bodies need it helps point you towards a good diet (and there are easy, tasty recipes to try throughout the book).

Starting To Get Fit

How fit are you? That's the first question to answer and Dr Rowan shows you an easy way to do this. He also highlights the general rules of how to get fit from making what you do fun, to the importance of exercising regularly.

Your Personal Fitness Programme

Keeping fit and looking in good shape is a very personal pastime. So in this part of the book *you* decide what you wish to achieve with an exercise programme and then work one out for yourself. Dr Rowan explains the range of exercises you need to include and then sets out a fitness chart for you to fill in and log yourself.

Stamina, Strength and Suppleness

These are the three ingredients of fitness. They're important and each is explained clearly with tips on how it can be developed, along with specific exercises designed to help you increase your own stamina, strength and suppleness.

Running, Jogging and Walking

Running, jogging and walking are at the heart of most activity sports so this section includes a personal 12-week jogging programme and advice on the right and wrong ways to set about it.

Sporting Life

'Sport should be fun,' says Dr Rowan but sadly a lot of people find it hard to stay fit because they pick activities that they don't really enjoy. Here he helps to put that right, looking at a wide range of sports and showing what each one will do for you in terms of developing overall fitness.

Looking Good

Looking good helps you feel good, so tips on hair care, skin care and looking after your teeth are just some of the ways of enjoying a healthy life.

Food and a Healthy Diet

We are lucky in the western world to have an abundance of food types and this should make it easy to eat a good, healthy and enjoyable diet. From explaining what a healthy diet really is, to a close look at what 'diets' and 'dieting' do to our bodies, and from a question and answer survey about how much you know about food and drink, to a look at the vitamins and minerals in the food we eat (or should eat), Dr Rowan shows all the advantages of eating the right balance of foods.

Body Wise is a positive book with a positive message. Life isn't all about pain and sacrifice and Dr Rowan shows that healthy living is about having fun, looking good, enjoying food and making friends.

Read it and find out for yourself.

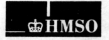 **HMSO**

HMSO publications are available from:

HMSO Publications Centre
(Mail, fax and telephone orders only)
PO Box 276, London, SW8 5DT
Telephone orders 071-873 9090
General enquiries 071-873 0011
(queuing system in operation for both numbers)
Fax orders 071-873-8200

HMSO Bookshops
49 High Holborn, London, WC1V 6HB
(counter service only)
071-873 0011 Fax 071-873 8200
258 Broad Street, Birmingham, B1 2HE
021-643 3740 Fax 021-643 6510
Southey House, 33 Wine Street, Bristol, BS1 2BQ
0272 264306 Fax 0272 294515
9-21 Princess Street, Manchester, M60 8AS
061-834 7201   Fax 061-833 0634
16 Arthur Street, Belfast, BT1 4GD
0232 238451 Fax 0232 235401
71 Lothian Road, Edinburgh, EH3 9AZ
031-228 4181 Fax 031-229 2734

HMSO's Accredited Agents
(see Yellow Pages)

and through good booksellers

Printed in the UK for HMSO
Dd 294791 c 100 9/92